THE PSYCHOLOGY OF
INTELLIGENCE AND WILL

Founded by C. K. Ogden

The International Library of Psychology

INDIVIDUAL DIFFERENCES
In 21 Volumes

I	The Practice and Theory of Individual Psychology	*Adler*
II	The Neurotic Constitution	*Adler*
III	Duality	*Bradley*
IV	Problems of Personality	*Campbell et al*
V	An Introduction to Individual Psychology	*Dreikurs*
VI	The Psychology of Alfred Adler and the Development of the Child	*Ganz*
VII	Personality	*Gordon*
VIII	The Art of Interrogation	*Hamilton*
IX	Appraising Personality	*Harrower*
X	Physique and Character	*Kretschmer*
XI	The Psychology of Men of Genius	*Kretschmer*
XII	Handreading	*Laffan*
XIII	On Shame and the Search for Identity	*Lynd*
XIV	A B C of Adler's Psychology	*Mairet*
XV	Alfred Adler: Problems of Neurosis	*Mairet*
XVI	Principles of Experimental Psychology	*Piéron*
XVII	The Psychology of Character	*Roback*
XVIII	The Hands of Children	*Spier*
XIX	The Nature of Intelligence	*Thurstone*
XX	Alfred Adler: The Pattern of Life	*Wolfe*
XXI	The Psychology of Intelligence and Will	*Wyatt*

THE PSYCHOLOGY OF
INTELLIGENCE AND WILL

H G WYATT

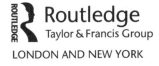

Routledge
Taylor & Francis Group

LONDON AND NEW YORK

First published in 1930 by
Routledge, Trench, Trubner & Co., Ltd.
2 Park Square, Milton Park, Abingdon, Oxfordshire OX14 4RN
711 Third Avenue, New York, NY 10017

First issued in paperback 2014

Routledge is an imprint of the Taylor and Francis Group, an informa business

British Library Cataloguing in Publication Data
A CIP catalogue record for this book
is available from the British Library

The Psychology of Intelligence and Will
ISBN 0415-21071-2
Individual Differences: 21 Volumes
ISBN 0415-21130-1
The International Library of Psychology: 204 Volumes
ISBN 0415-19132-7

ISBN 13: 978-1-138-87545-6 (pbk)
ISBN 13: 978-0-415-21071-3 (hbk)

CONTENTS

PAGE

PREFACE vii

PART I

I. THE QUEST FOR INTELLIGENCE . . . 3

II. THE STIMULUS-RESPONSE VIEW OF
INTELLIGENCE 14

III. THURSTONE ON INTELLIGENCE . . . 26

IV. THE GESTALT CONCEPT OF INTELLIGENCE . 32

V. THE FACULTY OF INTELLIGENCE . . 38

VI. THORNDIKE ON INTELLIGENCE . . . 58

VII. INTELLIGENCE AND SPEARMAN'S ' G ' . . 80

PART II

VIII. INTELLIGENCE AND INSTINCT . . . 101

IX. INTELLIGENCE THE MASTER OF INSTINCT . 120

PART III

X. PROBLEM OF INTELLIGENCE AND VOLITION 133

XI. FREE WILL AND A SCIENCE OF PSYCHOLOGY 160

XII. IS VOLITION UNIQUE ? 176

XIII. REPRESENTATIVE MODERN TREATMENTS OF
VOLITION 201

XIV. CONCLUSION AND SUMMARY . . . 239

REFERENCES AND NOTES 247

INDEX 271

v

PREFACE

THIS essay is the child (may it not prove also the parent) of disappointment. For some quarter of a century the author had been mainly occupied in the direct study not of psychology but of education, that is in applying (or misapplying) psychological principles. The attempt to derive enlightenment from books on the psychology of education still left him in important respects a purblind leader of the blind. To educate one must know not only how to impart knowledge, but how to train intelligence, how to regulate passion and therefore how to develop and strengthen will. Hence the ever insistent problem of the interplay of passion, intelligence and will, in the tangle of human mentality—a fascinating problem which induced a more serious reference to psychology for its solution. Then came the disappointment. Though to understand the conversion of the child as he is into the adult as he should be, a helpful theory of intelligence and volition is fundamental, professional psychology proved singularly unhelpful. Mostly it cared, or seemed to care, for neither of these things. Psychology of recent years has become more and more experimental, and interest is largely scattered on a multitude of experiments on details of behaviour, diverting attention from human behaviour as a whole. But even the ' general ' psychologist, when he comes to intelligence and volition turns strangely irrelevant or delusive. There is much measuring of intelligence, but few attempts to fathom it, and will is apt to be disposed of by treating it as something else.

The present essay purports to be a reasoned protest against this practice of disparagement, to challenge the assumptions,. and to expose the habits of thought which account for it, and to examine typical recent instances of belittlement or disregard of intelligence and will in psychology, and to suggest a more adequate and helpful view of them. Most of its chapters have been submitted to a few professional and lay acquaintances, and have received generally encouragement and appreciation. But one merciless critic has invalidated its contents mainly on the grounds that no attempt has been made to review, as each topic is treated, the previous experimental literature, or to base the position taken up on available or *ad hoc* experimental evidence. But inasmuch as the essay itself implicitly challenges these ' scientific ' conventions, and claims that one may say something useful in the present without first burdening the reader with epitomes of the past, it is left to the reader to settle whether this rejoinder has been justified.

I wish to express my thanks to Professor J. H. Muirhead (of the University of Birmingham) for considering chapters dealing with volition ; to Professor E. C. Tolman (of the University of California) and Professor E. S. Conklin (of the University of Oregon) for criticisms and helpful suggestions ; to Professor L. M. Terman (of Stanford University) for invaluable detailed advice ; to my friend Mr. A. S. Gibb for stimulating and suggestive discussions on topics to which the essay gave rise ; and to Professor A. E. Bott (of the University of Toronto) for his many invigorating comments.

PART I

INTELLIGENCE AND WILL

CHAPTER I

THE QUEST FOR INTELLIGENCE

IF there are two strictly psychological topics which would seem to a practical layman of most importance to investigate in his daily intercourse with his fellow men, one would be the topic of intelligence and the other that of character. Yet the science of psychology which has entered so many new fields in the last half and even quarter century, and is rapidly proving its utility in the practical guidance of life, has so far failed to give any adequate or coherent account of either of them.

The purpose of the first part of this work is to attempt an examination of the subject of intelligence, than which no topic or branch in psychology would seem at first sight to have been more indifferently and ineffectually treated, at any rate since psychology set about emancipating itself from speculative philosophy and claimed for itself recognition as a science.

There are of course reasons for this neglect. One of them lies in the very nature of intelligence itself. It courts obscurity. Others lie in the circumstances in which the *science* of psychology has been growing up : in the manner of its inception.

In fact it is the very claim of psychology to be a science, and therefore to pursue scientific methods, that has diverted psychologists from a systematic *theoretical* study of intelligence. The employment and

3

the refinement of the experimental methods of the physical sciences has opened up so many new fields and has been so promising of results that psychologists have been following the line of readiest experiment. The claims of psychology to the title of a science might thus be vindicated. For the same reason there has been a considerable reluctance to deal with aspects of psychology which do not lend themselves to objective and experimental treatment, and an accompanying distrust of unscientific introspective methods. Should it turn out that the nature of intelligence can, in the last analysis, be disclosed only by introspective methods, that would provide one reason why it has been so little understood. Introspection has been out of fashion : the tendency has been to neglect rather than to improve it as a method of psychological study.

Again, by a rather curious vicissitude of fortune, the modern evolutionary approach in psychology has helped to belittle intelligence. For the explanation of human behaviour has been sought first by way of the body (physiology) and then by way of the animal lower than man (animal and comparative psychology) rather than by an investigation of it at a stage of development where the functioning of intelligence is most in evidence.

Whatever light the physiological study of psychology— the study of the bodily accompaniments of mental process—has thrown upon the phenomena of sensation and perception, and the lower levels of behaviour, it is less illuminative of the higher thought processes. Yet in accordance with the human tendency to be prejudiced by the nature of one's occupations, the claim has been made that psychological phenomena are explicable in physiological terms, and psychological systems have actually been founded upon that basis. When we come to the higher thought processes, reflection and reasoning, physiological methods can be at best but supplementary to introspection : only introspection can disclose consciousness to consciousness. What goes on in the mind (whether above or below the conscious level) when we reason or reflect or attack intellectual problems, is not to be disclosed by examinatian of neural and cortical processes, but is observable only by looking within to see. Consequently intelligence has been either ignored or belittled by the physiological psychologist or evidence of it sought where it is least directly expressed. It is denied existence or significance as a distinctive psychological category.

The animal psychologist's treatment of intelligence has been somewhat different. One early consequence of the spread of evolutionary doctrines was the tendency to seek for evidence of human intelligence in the lower animals, for it was recognized that animal and human life was continuous, and that life in its lower stages contained the promise of man. The hoped for evidence was accordingly forthcoming, but its variety and abundance were in inverse proportion to its reliability.[1] Besides, the question arose why if animals performed the intelligent feats that were ascribed to them, their ordinary everyday achievements remained so modest. A brief era of faith and of travellers' tales about animal intelligence was succeeded by an age of scepticism and experiment.[2] There was a swing of the pendulum from one extreme to the other. In 1893 Lloyd Morgan announced his canon of parsimony,[3] a timely caution against the premature exaltation of the animal, and a few years later Thorndike in America was busy demonstrating the mechanical nature of the so-called intelligence of cats. But the downfall of the animal carried with it the downfall of man—for man is only the animal in a later stage of development ; and if intelligence in the animal is illusory, must not intelligence in man be illusory also ? Romanes had attempted to raise the animal to the human level : Thorndike retorted by reducing man to the animal.[4]

But some investigators have not stopped at the animal. Impelled by ' scientific ' conceptions and a desire for parsimony to render all human process in terms of its minima, there have not been wanting psychologists with still more radical aims. For if man is psychologically explicable in terms of the higher animal, by the same token the animal is psychologically explicable in terms of the lowlier animals, and ultimately the organic in terms of the inorganic. Man is not an animal, he is a machine.[5] Not only intelligence, but even consciousness itself has been denied him, or has been admitted as a noteworthy but useless phenomenon, like the beauty of a rose or the endless shimmer of the sea.

But to represent these as the sole reasons for the misunderstanding of intelligence would be misleading. There have always been and always will be psychologists primarily interested in a direct study of human nature, and neglectful of no method—including introspection— that may throw any light upon their subject. But even in their case intelligence has received meagre and inadequate attention.

Three reasons in particular may be suggested for their neglect of it. One is the aggrandisement of instinct (or of original endowment) and the keenness of the controversies which that topic has aroused. Another is the modern reaction against an intellectualist, and especially a faculty, psychology. A third reason is that it has been found perfectly practicable to deal with the products of intelligence, and even, presumably, to measure intelligence itself without a systematic enquiry into the nature of the process or function that was being measured. A word on each of these reasons.

The recognition of the place of instinct, or of original endowment, in human nature has been primarily due to the interest in animal psychology itself, for here, of course, instinctive behaviour is unmistakably exhibited But instinctive behaviour is far less evident in man, and yet it is clear that there must be some starting point of common characteristics from which individual human development takes off. No one now-a-days, not even the most extreme environmentalist, accepts the doctrine of the mere blank sheet. The mind is not just an inert recipient of impressions from without.

But once we admit that the environment and the individual organism co-operate in determining the individual's development, the question arises of their respective contributions. The controversy about instinct is in the main a controversy as to the kind and extent of the organism's share in the matter. The interest and antagonisms which this problem has engendered has diverted attention from the equally important problem of the nature of intelligence.

And with prejudice to the solution of the problem of instinct itself ; since, as will be contended later, the two factors in human behaviour are complementary, and one must have some understanding of their nature in order to delimit their respective spheres.

Illustrative of the failure adequately to recognize this fact was the symposium published in the *British Journal of Psychology* in 1910 professedly on the subject of the relation of Instinct to Intelligence ; in which the five contributors devoted the bulk of the argument to an analysis of the concept of instinct, and disposed of intelligence in vague or general terms.[6] This emphasis upon instinct has been accentuated by the progress of abnormal psychology, for as abnormalities are ascribable (or at any rate ascribed) more often to the mishandling of instinctive demands than to anything else, psychopathology has been largely concerned in an elaborate investigation of instinctive drives and urges. This reference of behaviour to instinct tends to obscure intelligence and to conceal its essential character.

Any realization of the essential nature of intelligence has been precluded also by another current prejudice— the fashionable (almost conventional) repudiation in psychological circles of anything savouring of a ' faculty.' The fallacy of the faculty psychology is claimed to have

been exploded.   The word faculty has become anathema.
To make serious use of it is to proclaim oneself out of
date.   But here again the pendulum may easily have
swung too far.   The true count against the faculties is
not that they do not exist, but that they do not exist
or function in the particular way that was claimed for
them, namely, as independent powers of the mind which
could be treated and developed in isolation from one
another, and the sum of which working together
constituted the mind in action.

But this is no reason for discarding the term altogether,
or for fighting shy of any suggestion that the mind has
distinguishable powers or capacities, so long as we
remember that in any concrete experience they are ever
affecting and conditioning one another.   It is unnecessary, it may indeed be even harmful, to substitute the
vaguer and less explicit term function, which implies
not an actual capacity, but only a use that may be served.
It may well be that the current preference for ' function '
prejudices clear thinking by the implication of a false
hypothesis ;   and if it turn out that faculty is a more
adequate description than function of the nature of
intelligence we have here a reason why the subject has
been avoided, or if considered, misconceived ' a priori.'
In seeking a function, it may well be that the *faculty* of
intelligence has been overlooked.

Lastly, we come to the contribution of the intelligence
testers.   With one or two exceptions, it might seem a
matter for surprise how little light they have so far shed
upon the essential nature of that intelligence they have
been so patiently and usefully measuring.   But when we
consider the circumstances of the test movement the
surprise vanishes.   The test movement has been a
typical illustration of the way in which a science builds
itself up.   Science begins with observations and experiments, and proceeds to theories and systems ;   and in
the process works out an experimental technique.   Its
incidental discoveries and generalizations are often of

practical human service, and when this service is clear and considerable, the formulation of theories attracts for the time being the less interest and attention.

Similarly in the case of the test movement the interest has been primarily practical, and as with improved technique the results of attempts at measurement have been proving of direct utility, interest has lain rather in improving methods and technique, and less in developing the theoretical aspects of the subject. The very success of the movement has been something of a hindrance to the systematic study of intelligence as such.

Though Binet, the pioneer of the movement, felt the need of some formulation of the concept before he had worked out his test scale, his discussion was unsystematic and incidental to his main enterprise.[7] And since his scale became widely known, and provided a point of departure for the extension of his methods, the psychologists of the movement have been so absorbed in the elaboration of tests and their results that their discussions of the nature of that which they presumed to be testing are incidental, tentative, and impressionistic rather than considered conclusions after careful analysis.

Nevertheless—and here psychology parallels the progress of other sciences—the results of experiment have prompted theoretical enquiry ; progress of tests and the accumulation of test results have provoked excursions into theory And naturally ; for, apart from the native curiosity of the human mind, the very business of selecting and arranging a test series, whether for testing general intelligence or some specific capacity, requires some analysis of the processes to be investigated, in order to provide for each a corresponding test.

Yet, again, this analysis can perhaps be evaded without mishap by the substitution of statistical for analytical comparisons, and by accepting more or less objective criteria of intelligence without theoretical analysis so long as the correlations come out satisfactorily. So long as the test results and the criteria tally

B

closely, but not too closely, no immediate demand for theoretical enquiry need arise—the interested public are being supplied with an instrument for measuring and comparing something it is useful to measure and compare. Moreover, it is just a set of agreed upon useful qualities that constitute the criterion itself. "This and that," says the teaching public, "is what we count as intelligence." "And this and that," reply the testers, "is what we measure. We present you accordingly with a trouble-saving device." Consequently there have not been wanting psychologists who have expressed no interest in the theoretical side of the subject.[8] They are satisfied that they can go on elaborating measuring instruments without it.

And indeed if that were all that the tests claimed for themselves their conclusion would be acceptable ; if, that is to say, they were merely economical expedients for enabling teachers or others to confirm their own opinions. But a difficulty arises when the tests are used to check and appraise the opinions of the teachers themselves. For here we have the tests claiming to supersede their own criteria. They are caught cutting away their own foundation, denying the validity of their own premises.

From this policy of suicide there are two opposite ways of escape. One is to seek safety in numbers. The criterion is not what these or those believe, but the common measure of the opinions of a great number. The obvious retort, however, that the few are wise and the many foolish next suggests the opposite alternative—the criterion shall be the verdict of the few wise judges. But here we are worse off than before ; for when we ask the experts what are the criteria of intelligence we find that they do not agree among themselves. "Quot homines tot sententiae." They nearly all express themselves differently. But the reason they differ is precisely that they have been content with a statistical treatment of their data, and have, with rare exceptions, undertaken no careful analytical study of the concept of intelligence itself.

So far, then, we have as our criteria only one opinion against another ; and so long as this is the case every teacher has a right to reject the findings of the testers with the retort that this is a free country, and "my opinion is as good as yours" ; and "I am as intelligent a judge of my students' intelligence as you are." If then the teacher expresses his surprise that his bright pupil A has been scored unduly low, and B unduly high by the tests, the testers have at present no right to gainsay him.

It is perhaps too much to hope that a single attempted analysis of intelligent process will suffice to present an authoritative criterion, but systematic analysis is at any rate the only way by which agreement will eventually be reached, and an authoritative criterion be set up to break the present vicious circle in which the testing is involved.

Typical of this disagreement amongst experts was the symposium on the meaning of the term intelligence published in 1921[9] to which no less than fourteen psychologists contributed. But the contributors as a whole were not answering the theoretical question. They were debating the question what it was that tests tested ; they were not first expounding a theory of intelligence, in order to see afterwards if the tests tested it. They were not concerned, that is to say, with investigating intelligence as a significant function of the mind, or with finding its place in the scheme of mental process or structure. Most of them contented themselves with a practical rather than a psychological answer. Intelligence is the organizing capacity, the capacity to learn, the capacity to adapt oneself to novel situations, the power of good responses in respect of truth or fact, adjustment to the environment, or the capacity for knowledge, and so on. Only one of them gave a psychological answer to a psychological question—

" intelligence is the capacity to carry on abstract or conceptual thinking." In this they were following the example set by early protagonists of measurement, Meumann, Stern, and Binet, who either defined intelligence in terms of its practical use, or at the most (Binet) as the functioning of one or more of a set of familiar mental processes.[10]   There was no hint of a possibility that they had before them a distinct mental category or property of the first importance, the analysis and explanation of which was cardinal to the development of psychology itself.   To the questions what is the mental quality which enables its possessor to adjust himself to his environment, to meet novel situations, to make good responses, or to acquire knowledge, or, for the matter of that, to think conceptually, better than B or C ; and how does it fit in with what else we know of mental qualities or processes, no answer was given.

This omission indicates the gap that so often exists between the psychologist at practice and the psychologist of theory. They are occupied in two universes of discourse, which they fail to relate to one another.   It would have been perfectly easy, for example, to have rendered adjustment to the environment, or to novel conditions, or the acquiring capacity, in terms of current psychology, for most text books of current psychology undertake to do this, some of them written by contributors to this very symposium.   But the deliverances at the symposium left the *psychological* curiosity of the reader unsatisfied.   To attempt to satisfy that curiosity is however the psychologist's business.   Accordingly some typical present-day accounts of the mental processes involved in acquiring the new, or in adjustment to novel conditions—that is, in intelligent activity— have now to be considered.   Should any of them prove satisfactory, there will be no need to add another to the number.

Three views of intelligence—the psychological process

underlying new acquisition, and adjustment to new situations—will be considered in turn, the views namely :

(1) Of the stimulus-response psychologist,
(2) Of a critic of that theory, Professor Thurstone,
(3) Of the Gestalt school of psychology.

CHAPTER II

THE STIMULUS-RESPONSE VIEW OF INTELLIGENCE

THE purpose of this chapter is to estimate the adequacy of the account of intelligence rendered by the stimulus-response psychologist. No attempt will be made to appraise the validity of the stimulus-response doctrine as a whole. Illustrative material will be taken from two recent works, F. H. Allport's *Social Psychology* and L. C. Bernard's books on *Instinct* and on *Social Psychology*, as typical exponents of the school.

It will be helpful to begin with the briefest possible resumé of the leading tenets of the doctrine.

Of three classes of factors or determinants in human behaviour the stimulus-response psychologist recognizes primarily two : the environment or objective stimuli, and the body of the organism, with certain neural mechanisms or inner behaviour patterns already pre-determined in its structure, and therefore entailing certain overt patterns of response. A third possible determinant, namely the Ego, or some separate power of the Ego to modify or change the innate behaviour patterns or to initiate innovations in behaviour, is denied influence in the matter, and consciousness or conscious processes are therefore also excluded.[1] In the forms of emotion, feeling, cognition, and conation, consciousness, an interesting accompaniment of behaviour, plays no part in determining it.

It must then be clearly understood that the term ' stimulus ' (objects or movements in the environment acting on a sense organ) excludes, by hypothesis, conscious content or process, though it includes ' in-body ' movements external to the nervous system, but capable of acting on afferent nerve endings.[2]   It is the stimuli that occasion the reaction or the situation (or complex of stimuli) that occasions the response.

In short, the environment (or sum of possible stimuli) takes one of the leading parts in the government and development of human behaviour.   The body is responsible for the other.   It is not to be regarded as a passive agent.   It begins life with certain behaviour patterns innate (or present from birth) or innately determined.   That is to say, there are certain groups of predominant or prepotent reflexes, or reactions to stimuli ; and these may appear overtly either as random movements, that is as reactions to no obvious external stimuli, or as definite types of reaction to definite types of stimuli, as when, for example, holding its head firmly provokes in the infant cries or screams, and stroking its cheek a smile.

Allport gives six groups of prepotent reflexes, starting and withdrawing, rejecting, struggling, hunger reactions, sensitive zone reactions, sex reactions.[3]   Bernard distinguishes tropisms, random movements, reflexes and instincts, instances of instincts (in his use of the term) being chains or complexes of reflexes controlling breathing, eating, digestion, and other internal processes.[4]   This is in contrast to complex behaviour habits frequently recognized as instincts, such for instance as those of Professors MacDougall, Colvin, and others, of which common examples are the gregarious instincts, instincts of flight and fear, instincts of self-assertion, family instincts, and so on.   It is neural mechanisms alone that can claim to be inherited, and these play the second role as determiners of human behaviour.

But, as the development of character and personality in the organism implies a continuity of changes or modifications in the original reflex endowment, the problem arises of accounting for these changes.   This problem is solved by referring to the two processes known as the conditioned reflex and trial-and-error.[5] If with a stimulus A which innately provokes a reaction there is repeatedly associated a new stimulus B, after a certain number of repetitions B will suffice by itself to provoke the reaction. Thus new situations come to occasion an old response. This is a case of a conditioned reflex ; the response has been conditioned to a new stimulus.

The question then remains how the responses may change, for development of behaviour consists very largely in changed responses. This problem is solved in terms of trial-and-error or rather of trial and success. The organism acquires new responses by the establishment of chance successes. The first innate reactions to stimuli, or responses to a situation, not being successful, others occur, and those successful tend to get fixed. It requires unusual stimuli (a new or unfamiliar situation), as Bernard points out, to start the processes.[6] As to the way in which the successful responses become established, Allport frankly admits there is no satisfactory explanation.[7]

The possible objection that the two processes do not seem to cover cases of thinking out a problem is met by the claim that thought will be found, on analysis, to be only trial-and-error in an abridged form on the ideational plane.[8]

On one point it is necessary to lay special stress, before considering the use made of the doctrine. It is cardinal to the doctrine that there shall be no third factor, in the form of consciousness or the Ego, determining the reactions. Allport is clear about this. " Consciousness exerts no influence and therefore explains nothing in mutual relations of human beings."[9] To admit a third factor is of course to abandon the position. It is true that the stimulus-response psychologist speaks of a loud sound, or of physical restraint, as stimuli arousing in the infant the reactions of fear or of anger. But we are bound by his premises to conclude

THE STIMULUS–RESPONSE VIEW 17

that though using, for convenience, popular forms of language, we have to abstract from the meaning any suggestion of consciousness in understanding what actually occurs. Thus if we exclude consciousness it is not the loudness of the sounds that provokes the infant to hide his face or to shrink, but the nervous impulses set up by the impinging of atmospheric energy upon his sense organ—it makes no difference whether he *hears* the sound or not. And when, again, the head of a newborn child is held tight so that the usual random movements are inhibited, it is not any anger at constraint that occasions the struggling and screaming that follow, but the holding of the head in this manner involves a number of objective stimuli which arouse nerve impulses that induce in the effectors the movements that we witness in struggling and screaming. It is not because he *feels* constrained that the infant struggles, but because his neural machinery necessitates the response.

As examples of stimuli Watson names " such things as rays of light of different lengths, sound waves differing in amplitude, length, phase, and combination, gaseous particles given off in such small diameters that they affect the membrane of the nose ; solutions which contain particles of matter of such size that the taste buds are thrown into action " and so on. This of course is consistent with his denial of the influence of consciousness ; and wherever a stimulus-response psychologist is found including consciousness, as for example perception, in the stimulus, he has admitted a third party in behaviour in spite of his disclaimer ; and has given no reason why it is to be admitted in the one case in defiance of his principles and excluded in others.[10]

The Application of the Stimulus-Response Doctrine to the Question of the Nature of Intelligence.

Where all mental development is explicable in terms of conditioned reflex or of trial-and-error, there is of

course no room for a separate functioning of intelligence
to affect behaviour for better or for worse.   Intelligence,
so far as it is recognized at all, can at best be a synonym
for successful conditionings or for successful 'trials.'
If A is more intelligent than B this can mean only that
A's successes in the trial-and-error processes are more
frequent than B's, or that the stimuli that condition
his reflexes are more favourable stimuli.   For if the
behaviour of the organism is determined by objective
stimuli it cannot at the same time be determined by a
capacity in the organism to solve its problems or adapt
its conduct to them.   If it exercises a capacity for
solving the problems of life, its behaviour is not determined chiefly by objective stimuli.   Thus in any given
situation, on the stimulus-response premise, there can
be in A or B no power as such of differentiating or
selecting between possible responses or of apprehending,
or adapting behaviour to, the requirements of the
situation.   One cannot at one and the same time
maintain that all one's behaviour is the result of stimuli
and also that some faculty or separate power called
intelligence affects it.   To accept the latter statement
is to abandon the former.   Consistently with the
stimulus-response tenets, then, intelligence if it means
anything can mean only a high proportion of chance
successes, successes not due to any special power or
initiative resident in the organism, but solely to the
effects of environmental stimuli upon its neural
organizations.   For what else can it signify and preserve
consistency ?

It is not therefore out of keeping with his general
position for Allport to declare intelligence to be a
servant, not a master, in his mechanical menage ; for
intelligent acts on the stimulus-response principle are
just as much determined by the stimuli as any others.
But it is rather less in keeping with it to select for its
master simply the autonomic activities.[11]   As successful
conditioning, or successful trials, there is no reason given

why any of the six prepotent reflexes should not equally claim intelligence when they function successfully.

But when in a later chapter of his book, we find him defining intelligence as the capacity for solving the problems of life—an ability which enables its possessor to advance beyond the stage of crude trial-and-error in overt manipulation of its objects to the use of symbol reactions, he is contradicting his own premises. No organism whose behaviour is determined by its environment can have a capacity to determine its own behaviour—to attack a problem in a better or worse way.

Moreover the premises have so far been disregarded that this capacity is said to comprise a " capacity for observation," " constructive imagination," and " sound judgment or the capacity for making a mature decision at a crisis."[12]   The stimulus-response doctrine admits of no such distinctive capacities. For at least two reasons.   One is that observation, constructive imagination, and sound judgment, are all highly conscious processes ; and by hypothesis these have no influence upon behaviour.   A second reason is that there is no room for these qualities to exert any influence in an organism completely dominated by objective stimuli.

Equally significant is Professor Bernard's difficulty in satisfactorily accounting for the place of intelligence in behaviour. After reaffirming his general position that the cortical mechanisms are dominated by environmental stimuli,[13] he makes the statement that " the cerebral cortex responding to stimuli from without must take the initiative in making new adjustment patterns demanded by a changing environment and in providing for the regular functioning of the old ones, including the organic mechanisms, because of the highly flexible and responsive character of its neural organization."[14] If his statement be taken at its face value, the intelligent reader encounters the following problems :

(1) How can the cortex be determined in its conduct

by environmental stimuli, and at the same time take the initiative ?

(2) Even assuming that the cortex takes the initiative, wherein does the power of the cortex reside ? Is it a capacity of the cortex to exercise its own initiative, or does the Ego exercise it through its conscious processes ?

If it is the cortex that takes the initiative, we are committed to the conclusion that the brain (as distinct from the mind) exercises choice ; but if the term cortex is used loosely for the mind or the Ego expressing itself through the cortex, then we have admitted a psychic determinant of behaviour in addition to the environment and the original neural mechanisms. In either case our author would have abandoned his leading principles, by claiming in opposition to them that in behaviour where cortical functions are involved (and this includes all conscious behaviour) something other than environmental stimuli determine the responses.

Suppose however we do not take his statement at its face value, but assume that the intention of the passage has been misconstrued. It is perhaps intended to suggest, not that the cortex has any initiating power of its own, but that objective stimuli in new combinations (that is, new situations) may provoke new reactions, and that this happens where cortical levels are engaged. It is the environment that initiates new behaviour, acting through the cortex. In this case, the only explanation that the stimulus-response psychology can consistently offer of intelligence is that it is chance success in conditioning or chance success in trial-and-error. From this position it follows that the intelligence level of the individual will be subject to fluctuations with changes in the environment, and only those who can command a continuously favourable environment over a prolonged period may be expected, for example, to show any consistency in their I.Q. And secondly if we translate intelligence by successful behaviour, and not by an inherent capacity as such, we are faced with the conclusion that a man is intelligent because he is successful, and not successful because he is intelligent. Moreover success is a relative term—it means different things to different people. To those who conceive success in terms of public usefulness, a philanthropist is *ipso facto* more intelligent than a scoundrel. To those who measure it by the dollar, the rich are *ipso facto* more intelligent than the poor, and the child who has inherited millions has the most innate intelligence of us all.

The stimulus-response psychologist would refuse, no doubt, to accept these implications of his doctrine. Indeed it is only because he conceals their implications that his principles can appear as plausible as they do. But they do not fail, all the same, to influence his conscious reasoning Bernard's argument seems to be a case in point. After considering the functions of the cortex in human behaviour, he comes to examine the nature and conditions of intelligence. " Intelligence," he says, " is the most significant of all the individual powers serving the adjustment of the organism to its environment. It is a very complex system of phenomena, embracing all sorts of adjustment capacities and techniques.''[15] Now ' adjustment ' belongs to that class of vague convenient words which can bear different meanings according to the requirements of the moment. In a sense, of course, we are adjusting to our environment all the time ; at least, we are always doing something in connection with it and because it is there. But to use it in this sense of intelligence is to make us all equally intelligent and on all occasions. By adjustment Bernard clearly means something more than this, and the additional meaning he appears to attach to it is precisely the only meaning which, as already contended, must attach to it in keeping with his premises : namely, that of success in effecting an object, whatever that object may be.

That this is his real criterion becomes still more apparent from his endorsement of a summary of

Professor Woodworth's of certain factors stated to be basic to intelligence.[16]   These comprise ' retentiveness,' " the power to apply what one learns and retains to other problems," " responsiveness to relationships," ' attention ' (in order to build up an effective attitude towards one's subject), ' persistence ' (we pronounce the flighty or inattentive person unintelligent because he appears to be incapable of mastering a situation or carrying anything through) ; " a certain degree of sub-missiveness or humility " (for a person too stubborn may try to do more than he can accomplish) ; curiosity (there can be no adequate orientation in behaviour without this quality) ; and alertness to new situations, to be able to sense our problems, to understand them, and then to solve them.

" These factors in intelligence," says Bernard, " are not concrete behaviour patterns, but they are synthetic attitudes towards behaviour patterns which count for effectiveness—another synonym for intelligence—in adjustment.   In other words it is not persistence or humility or alertness, but the readiness or ability to persist or be humble or alert that are some of the basic factors in intelligence."[17]

Yet a mere glance at this list will show that it is not intelligence that is being described at all, but a number of factors, by no means implied in intelligence, that (sometimes even in spite of unintelligence) contribute to success.   I am not necessarily intelligent because I have a good memory (some mental defectives have good memories) ; I may think or work intelligently and yet be weak in recall ; I may be humble and intelligent or humble and unintelligent ; again, I may be intelligent, self-confident and persistent ; or I may be intelligent enough, but fail of success through lack of persistence or even lack of curiosity, and so on.

Of course these factors or qualities will assist the intelligent person to make his intelligence more effective, in other words will help him to succeed, but to call them basic factors to intelligence itself is to defy common experience, without justifying the defiance. In fine, just as the stimulus-response psychology has no place in its explanation of human nature or behaviour for emotion or consciousness, so it has no place for intelligence, which it can deal with only by treating it as something else.

Professor Bernard indeed is led to commit himself further by exaggerating in connection with intelligence the significance of incentives or drives. We may admit, of course, that where there is drive, incentive, motivation (Bernard does not here define his terms, but they seem to imply some strength of impulse towards action or consciousness of some object as worth attaining) successful behaviour is the more likely to follow. But the conclusion that " many times the chief distinction between an intelligent and an unintelligent child or adult lies in the degrees of incentive which actuate them "[18] does not follow from the premises. The chief distinction between the children is obviously in their degrees of intelligence ; and, as for this corresponding closely with degree of drive, so far is this from being the case that it often happens that the more intelligent of two persons may exhibit the less drive of the two, as where in doing mechanical work calling for little intelligence the more intelligent individuals work with less drive than their fellows, and do worse work. That the highly intelligent pupil in an ordinary class tends to do relatively inferior work through lack of competition in spite of his intelligence is a recognized reason for the institution of special classes for bright children ; and investigations in industrial psychology have shown that workers rating high in intelligence tests are found doing worse work than less intelligent fellow workers through greater boredom, that is, through lack of drive.[19] Here then we have another example of the confusion of intelligence with other factors that make for success in one's work or occupation. But then this confusion of intelligence with success is inherent in the stimulus-response psychology.

Allport's and Bernard's treatment of the subject illustrates the one insuperable difficulty which all mechanistic psychologies encounter in explaining human conduct on its higher level. They are committed by their postulates to a denial, or at least an ignoring, of the very data which it is the prime business of psychology to explain ; namely, ordinary human experience and behaviour. To the unsophisticated and unpsychological human his conscious processes and his emotions make all the difference in his behaviour. In ordinary life, as expressed in ordinary language, we are moved by anger, or roused by curiosity ; a sudden pain causes us to flinch ; the loss of a dear one distresses us ; a joke makes us laugh. Almost every thought we think and every sentence we speak is couched in language which assumes (as its users assume) the influence upon the behaviour of each of us of our thoughts and emotions. As distinct from the physical sciences, human psychology concerns itself with just those human phenomena which are commonly explained and described in emotional and 'conscious' terms—the relations of human beings to one another.

Amongst the predominantly 'human' phenomena which have thus to be disregarded is that which passes under the name of intelligence, as a quality or capacity inherent in A or B, and inherent in greater degree in one than the other, of using effectively, in virtue of that inherent quality, and turning to account for his own purpose, elements in his environment. To the stimulus-response psychologist the expression " to use one's intelligence " is necessarily meaningless ; as is the common judgment of this or that person or piece of conduct being more intelligent than another.

And as with consciousness and emotions, the dilemma has to be faced of either admitting their significance and abandoning the doctrine, or of maintaining the doctrine and being unable to explain how, if they serve no purpose in human life, they come to be there.

So with intelligence. How is it if intelligence has no distinctive meaning we actually do draw a distinction at all between acts which are intelligent and those which are not, and do not assimilate it merely to chance success ? To this question it is the business of psychology to provide an answer. To this the stimulus-response psychologist has no consistent answer to give.

C

CHAPTER III

THURSTONE ON INTELLIGENCE

In sharp contrast with the doctrine just considered is the account of intelligence given in his book on the subject by Dr. Thurstone.[1] In human behaviour the objective simulus is strictly subordinate. The prime mover is the inner urge. In fact, each piece of human behaviour—the psychological process, as Thurstone calls it—is a series of stages in the progress from the urge to its satisfaction. For all mental process starts with the unrest of the inner self, and ends with its contentment. Thought is a part of the process : it can thus be described as half finished conduct. The objective stimulus figures as a mere instrument of the urge. The organism seeks for stimuli in order to provide a means of satisfaction ; they are subordinate directors rather than initial prompters of action. Thurstone analyses the psychological act or process into several stages, which may however be compressed into the following :[2]

(1) The experience of the urge.
(2) The seeking for suitable stimuli.
(3) Action in relation to the stimuli.
(4) Satisfaction of the urge.

In this simple scheme it is not difficult to find a place for intelligence. It figures, as we might expect, as a conscious process intermediate between the urge and its satisfaction. But the word intermediate needs qualification, for as regards the degree of intelligence it is all important just where the conscious direction takes place. Intelligence consists in ideation or reflection at the earliest point in the process after the experience

26

of the impulse.   In other words, Thurstone makes the position which the ideation occupies in the series a criterion of the degree of the intelligence.   Intelligence is the capacity to make impulses focal (that is, to bring them into full consciousness) at their early unfinished stage of formation.[3] For the earlier the point, or the further the distance from the overt act, at which the impulse is made focal, the greater the range of possible actions.

Since intelligence involves making impulse focal early, it follows that the process is inhibitory, for it is obvious that instead of acting immediately on impulse there is a check of the impulse, in order to interpose reflection. Intelligence is thus a capacity to inhibit instinct at an early stage of its functioning.[4] The actual process of intelligent thinking at this stage is characterized as ideational trial-and-error.[5]

A simple instance of the psychological process would be the following :

I feel hungry (the urge).   But instead of seizing the first bit of bread that comes handy, I consider the best way to satisfy my hunger (intelligence, ideational trial-and-error), and seek for food (the stimulus), which I then consume (the overt act), and am satisfied ; there is contentment of the inner self ; or as Thurstone puts it, " there is quiescence at the energy source." The urge is satisfied.

On this account of the nature of intelligence the following comments seem justified :

Assuming that the psychological sequence from initial urge to overt act is the universal or even the typical mental process, it is surely not true that reflection and intelligent reflection are limited in any way to one point in the process.   To take the example already given, in which the hungry man satisfies his craving. Surely one can ' ideate ' at any point along the line : in choosing the food, in cooking it, in laying it on the table, and in selecting which bits to eat and in which order.

And surely, secondly, I can reflect equally effectively whether the point at which I reflect is early or late in the proceedings, and equally ineffectively. I may, for instance, choose the wrong food ; I may then lay it inconveniently on the table, and I may or may not fail to secure for myself the best bits. It is difficult to see how the intelligence of the thinking depends in any way on the position of the thinking act at a particularly early, indeed at any special, place in the psychological process. It is no doubt true, as Thurstone points out, that if when aware of an impulse or an urge one stops to think instead of acting precipitately, one gives oneself scope for reflection, and therefore for variability of action ; but the thinking may be of a high or a low order of intelligence, and the stopping to think may or may not be due to intelligence.

Nor indeed is the making of the impulse focal at an early stage a particular sign of intelligence, as Thurstone also contends it is. After all, to make the impulse of hunger focal is only to be clearly aware that one is hungry. It is difficult to believe that there is anything noticeably intelligent about that awareness. Yet that is just the kind of awareness that does occur at the earliest stage, namely, the consciousness of a certain need.

In short, the intelligence or the degree of intelligence of my conduct does not consist in my reflecting just after the impulse, much less in my attending to the impulse (making it focal), nor yet in my having a larger number of possible actions to choose from. It lies rather in my manner of choice, in a certain capacity to choose effectively, and that capacity I may exercise on any topic that occurs, and at any point in the series.

But the further question arises whether the act sequence as Thurstone describes it is typical. Is the psychological process or sequence of ' urge-ideation-stimulus-overt-act-satisfaction ' the ordinary sequence ? Take the case, for example, in which A hits B, and B gets angry and returns the blow.   Does the matter really and usually begin with A feeling an urge of anger, seeking (perhaps after intelligent ideation, noticing that B is smaller than he is, etc.) a stimulus in B, and proceeding to satisfy his urge by pummelling B ?   And does B in this case begin by feeling the urge, rather than by feeling it in response to the stimulus imparted by A ?

Take another case : I see candy, feel greedy, buy it, and eat.   Can it reasonably be argued that the psychological process begins here with the urge, rather than with the perception of the candy ?   And as for the intelligence involved, the most scope for intelligence seems to come not at the beginning of the series, but in determining the greatest delight I can achieve for the least expenditure, namely after the percept and in one of the stages of the overt act.

Or again, a strange sight provokes my wonder, and I investigate it.   Here again the stimulus comes first, and such intelligence as is called for appears to be likely to display itself in the manner of investigating the object of wonder, namely during the overt act.

Finally it should be noticed that Thurstone gives three criteria of intelligence without attempting a comparative evaluation of them, so that one is left in doubt as to which is the most significant.   Intelligence is

(a) focalising early,

(b) inhibiting impulse ; and

(c) trial-and-error on the ideational plane.

He appears to give preference to (a), but we are left uncertain.   (b) clearly confuses intelligence with character, or with volition.   To inhibit an impulse, that is, to stop and not immediately satisfy my impulse indicates character at least as much as intelligence.   He who checks his impulse most is not therefore the most intelligent ; all that he does is to give his intelligence a chance to work at one useful point amongst others.   But a person of impulse may be and often is just as intelligent as a person of self-control.   In stating (c) that intelligence is ideational trial-and-error, Thurstone is not propounding a fresh thesis of his own ; he merely takes this description of intelligence from current peychology, and makes no attempt to justify it.   The position has already been contested in the previous chapter ; and the arguments against regarding the trial-and-error hypothesis as adequate apply just as cogently whether the trials take place in fact or only in imagination, for the two arguments are identical.

Lastly, the solecism is committed of confusing a general tendency to action with a universal idea.[6]   In Thurstone's opinion the earlier in the proceedings after the occurrence of the urge one becomes aware of the impulse the more universal is the corresponding concept.   It would seem that to be clearly aware of an impulse is an instance of a peculiarly intelligent grade of concept.   Whereas it is merely to be aware of an impulse and implies the lowest level of abstraction.   So much is Thurstone intrigued by this peculiar phantasy that we find him concluding his book with the suggestion that ability to focalize at a still earlier stage, if that were possible, in fact to do without focalization by proceeding immediately from the initiating urge, would be a peculiar mark of genius.[7] But this is to obliterate the distinction between the genius and the brute.

The doctrine of the stimulus and Thurstone's doctrine of the urge as universal determiner of action have this in common : they both exaggerate the significance of one of the factors in the situation, and both proceed from that exaggeration to a mechanical and artificial scheme, inconsistent with the facts of common experience. Both equally ignore the important third factor as a distinctive and significant factor, intelligence itself. Both regard the thinking process as a process of trial-and-error, thus denying it any intelligence in the ordinary acceptation of the term.   To both, intelligence as intelligence is illusion.

But there is one difference of importance between

these two standpoints. In the case of the stimulus theory intelligence is necessarily an illusion : it cannot be otherwise, consistently with the initial premises. But Thurstone's account of intelligence does not follow necessarily from the original premise of the urge, still less does his doctrine of intelligence as ideational trial-and-error. As will be contended later, though intelligence as a human experience is incompatible with a mechanical account of it, it is not by any means inconsistent with the experience of impulses or urges. Indeed, it may well be questioned whether it would function at all without them.

CHAPTER IV

THE GESTALT CONCEPT OF INTELLIGENCE

THE two views just examined agree in interpreting the 'intelligent' process as one of trial-and-error, whether overt (as in acquiring new skills) or ideational (in acquiring new knowledge). In striking contrast with this is a view of the mental process underlying adjustment to novel conditions, which is next to be considered, the view of an act of insight as a 'configuration' or 'Gestalt.'

A typical exposition of the Gestalt principle is available for English readers in *The Growth of the Mind*, by K. Koffka, a principle abundantly exemplified from experimental observations in W. Köhler's *The Mentality of Apes*, also in the present Library.

With the material supplied by these books as a basis, it is proposed to examine the adequacy of the principle of Gestalt to account for the facts.

Reasons have already been given for rejecting the trial-and-error hypothesis as inadequate, so that there is no need to supplement them with Koffka's criticisms of the same hypothesis included in his elaborate and searching examination of Thorndike's 'cat' experiments recorded in his book.[1] We may begin therefore by indicating important points in which the two hypotheses contrast.

In the trial-and-error view the new achievement or acquired performance is (a) a summation or series of 'successful' items ; (b) successful in the first instance according to the ordinary laws of chance or probability ; with (c) a tendency for the more frequent movements, or the more recent, to recur in virtue of this frequency or recency, or for the successful performance to be "stamped in" by pleasure or satisfaction. According to the principle of Gestalt the successful performance is not an aggregate of items, but a connected and inter-related whole ; the achievement is not a result of chance but an outcome of ' insight ' ; and is both attained and confirmed as a result of this ' insight,' and not mainly through the effects of frequency or accompanying pleasure.

In a typical case of learning the animal does not, to use popular language, hit on the right performance, still less, repeat it, by accident, he does so rather by grasping the situation, more or less suddenly.

This grasping the situation, or act of insight, calls for further analysis. The Gestalt psychology represents it as configurative, a configuration being in the words of Koffka " a coexistence of phenomena in which each member carries every other, and in which each member possesses its peculiarity only by virtue of and in connection with all the others."[2] Applied to a learned achievement it may be expressed as a performance whole, in which each part of the performance takes its place and its character from the whole.

How, then, does this act of insight come about ? What are the characteristics of the process ? A study of the performances of Köhler's apes in carefully designed experimental situations, and of Koffka's discussion of the subject, brings out the following points of interest.

The ' solution ' or the successful performance is noticeably different in several important respects from the movement series or performances which precede it. In the first place the parts of it are different, in the second their sequence is unique, and thirdly, the performance is marked by a smoothness, continuity, and certainty or confidence absent in the preceding hesitating and ineffective ' trial ' performances.. There is a fourth difference to be mentioned later.

Let us consider the following illustration :

A tempting bait or objective in the shape of bananas is placed outside and at some distance from the bars of the apes' cage. On the ground inside the cage is a stick too short to reach and draw in the banana even when used with the arm extended. But to one side of the objective and near enough to the bars to be drawn in by use of the short stick is a much longer stick.

In solving this problem an animal begins by trying to reach the objective with the short stick, and fails. The solution involves a different set of movements, namely first using the short stick to bring in the longer one, and then the longer one to bring in the banana. Yet several apes effect the solution, and though their reactions were not in every case sudden, yet the first successful performance meant the employment of many movements not previously made—the pushing of the longer stick through the bars.

To quote Köhler : " Sultan tries to reach the fruit with the smaller of the two sticks. Not succeeding, he tears at a piece of wire that projects from the netting of his cage, but that too is in vain. Then he gazes about him : (there are always, in the course of these tests some long pauses, during which the animals scrutinize the whole visible area). He suddenly picks up the little stick, once more goes to the bars, directly opposite to the long stick, scratches it towards him with the auxiliary, seizes it, and goes with it to the point opposite to the objective, which he secures."[3] The solution, or successful performance, it will be noted, here involves a set of movements different from those of the previous trials, arranged in an order of their own, and carried out with continuity and lack of hesitation in spite of their being the first of their kind.

To continue the quotation : " From the moment that his eyes fall upon the long stick, his procedure forms one consecutive whole, without hiatus, and, although the angling of the bigger stick by means of the smaller is an action that could be distinct and complete in itself, yet observation shows that it follows, quite suddenly, on an interval of hesitation and doubt—staring about—which undoubtedly has a relation to the final objective, and is immediately merged in the final action of the attainment of this end goal."

A fourth feature of these achievements is also significant. The repetition of the successful performances is not just a mere repetition. There are differences in detail. The animal may begin the performance from a different position in the cage, may seize a different part of the stick, or poke it through a different but equally serviceable pair of bars, and so on. But there is preserved in the successful performances the same pattern or structure—the pattern, namely, which fits the situation. The essential features of the solution are maintained.

Performances of this type are said to be effected with insight, and to betoken intelligence.

In applying the same principle to human intelligent acts it is of course unnecessary to design special experiments. Common experience can supply abundant instances. In the case of the two-stick problem itself, it is obvious that any child, not yet accustomed to estimating measurements of length, would be likely to follow the ape's behaviour. He would try to reach the objective with the handy stick, and failing with that, would notice the long stick and do as the ape did. On the same principle acts the boy, who wants to reach an apple on a branch above his reach. He begins, we will say, by jumping at it ; finds this to fail, and tries to climb the tree. The trunk is too smooth for him ; he desists ; takes a look around ; his eye lights upon a bench not far off ; he brings it, sets it under the branch, steps on it, and secures the apple. His observation of the bench was followed by " a reconstruction of the situation " ; and if he wanted to get another apple from the same position another time, his performance would preserve the same pattern, though it would differ in inessential details.

Such procedures, and they abound in human life, constitute a refutation of the trial-and-error hypothesis from the mere facts of the case themselves. The achievement is not a mere summation or stringing together of previous isolated items, and the items which make it up are not determined by frequency or recency or any particular serial position of the movements.

But the question which concerns us here is not, whether the new hypothesis is a more accurate statement of the facts, but whether it gives an adequate account of the nature of that intelligence to the existence of which it testifies.

Reasons for giving a negative answer to this question have already been suggested elsewhere.[4] They may be here summarized as follows :

The use of the metaphor Gestalt or configuration or structure does not help us to understand what the intelligent process is. We observe, and admit, its objective results, the set of movements which are configurative, but we are not helped by the outward patterned performance to understand or to conjecture what corresponding to it goes on in the mind. We await a psychological account of a psychological phenomenon.

The metaphor, so far as it goes, is actually misleading. It misplaces the emphasis. For, so far as it implies anything about the nature of intelligence at all, it certainly implies that it consists in effecting configurations. But a particular configuration may on any occasion be right or wrong, may or may not fit the situation or meet the requirement. To make configuration the criterion of intelligence misses the point, for it does not help us to distinguish between insight and illusion, a genuine grasp of the situation and error.

Configurations without sufficient insight are unfortunately extremely common in human life ; and account, when they are adhered to, for many disastrous errors of conduct. Every fresh hypothesis that we frame, whether about a momentary practical situation or whether for pure knowledge, constitutes a fresh configuration, a new shaping of the presented data, but it may be an intelligent or an unintelligent reading of the situation. Of two children approximately equal in age and experience most of us would credit with the greater insight the one who given a screw-driver and a board with a screw in it used the screw-driver to unscrew the screw than the one who used it to prise the screw off the board. But both have configured the situation. The mere act of configuration then does not account for the intelligence of the act. Our main question is thus left unanswered by the configuration theory.

If it be claimed that by configuration is meant a shaping of the situation in accordance with its needs, we may admit the emendation, but then we seem justified in claiming that the configuration metaphor is at least an unfortunate one, in that it suggests a wrong emphasis, in fact, that it has " misconfigured itself." For it has left out the most important feature from the picture, which is, not the configuration as such, but its relevancy.

But even granting the amendment, we have still to consider how this alteration of conduct to fit the situation takes place, in a word, how the organism adjusts to a novel situation ; what mental process in fact does intelligence imply. To this the theory offers no answer. But it is the business of the psychologist to attempt to find one.

CHAPTER V

THE FACULTY OF INTELLIGENCE

It follows from the reasoning of the preceding chapter that the Gestalt contribution to our subject lies not in solving the problem of intelligence but in having restated it more correctly. The new performance, the concrete adjustment to a novel situation, appears on analysis not a series of instinctive or previously acquired separate activities, but—a new performance. Not, of course, that it is entirely new, it is not an act of spontaneous creation, but it is new in the sense that the pattern or arrangement of the constituent elements is a new pattern, and these elements are newly modified to suit the pattern of the whole. Köhler's apes were of course already accustomed to move their arms and legs and handle objects and so on, but particular selections and modifications of these movements were involved in adapting them to the new pattern or the fresh construction of the situation ; and here their insight is assumed to lie.

Where the Gestalt account of the matter appears to err is in making the configuration or pattern as such a criterion of intelligent behaviour, and not in pursuing the analysis further. After all, there are configurations and configurations. The boy who for the first time tries to reach his apples by climbing the tree, and falls, has undoubtedly effected a configuration : he has patterned the situation in such a way that his consequent series of movements constitutes a performance whole, and every item is there as part of that performance. He has not just put together a set of random instinctive activities. Each movement of body, arm, and leg is

38

adapted to fit the situation as constructed. But he does not get the apple. His brother, surveying the scene with him, effects a different configuration. His configuration or pattern includes the fetching of a bench and a stick, standing on the bench beneath the apple and knocking it down with the stick. If insight is synonymous with configuration as such, the one boy showed as much insight as the other and his act was as intelligent as the other's. And all newly patterned behaviour must be equally indicative of intelligence; irrespective of whether it solves the problem, meets the novel situation, or not.

If, on the other hand, the term configuration be restricted to such a patterning of the situation as solves the problem, and to no other, two objections to the configuration doctrine arise. One is that it employs a misleading and confusing metaphor, which implies that the *patterning* is the test of insight; the other—which is the crucial one—that it does not explain wherein resides the psychological superiority in insight of a pattern that solves the problem over any other. But it is just this that constitutes the problem of intelligence itself. The doctrine thus ignores the heart of the problem it has set out to solve. It leaves intelligence unaccounted for.

The Gestalt psychologist has told only half of the story, he has brought it to the point where it invites continuation and has not continued it. A reason why he has observed this limitation is not difficult to suggest. He has come to the problem of intelligence already committed to his Gestalt hypothesis in general, a hypothesis derived and applied in other fields, and is satisfied when he discovers that the same principle again applies. Indeed to pursue the analysis further might be found to endanger the validity of this principle. Moreover it is one of his own assumptions that a configuration is an ultimate unit of mental structure, so that further analysis is not even warranted.

But the disinterested enquirer is free to pursue the matter further. Nor is his path particularly arduous. The question wherein lies the difference between intelligent and unintelligent configuration can be answered by a reference to the behaviour of the apes as observed and recorded by Köhler.

Köhler's experiments consisted in setting his apes a series of practical problems—how to attain an objective attainable not by going directly for it ; but only by discovering indirect means. Though therefore the impulse which perception of the object prompted initiated the various indirect performances it was not of itself sufficient to account for their nature and composition. For all that an impulse *qua* impulse can do is to impel the organism in the direction of its goal. It provides the ' drive ' only. We cannot therefore in terms of impulse account for the apes' mastery of indirect approaches to their objectives, still less of the particular ' configurative ' approaches of which they proved themselves capable. But we can seek an explanation of them in the ape's relation not to the mere impulse which starts his excitement but to the objective to which it is directed. Of this objective the ape was surely aware, for he is reported constantly attending to it ; and his movements are constantly in the same general direction. He was in fact endeavouring to reach his goal. In other words the configurations which he achieved were configurations in relation to a conscious objective, and determined by that consciousness. But this is to allow that it was not the configuration that constituted the essence of the achievement, but the configuration-in-relation-to-the-objective.

Moreover, if the objective were not the deciding factor, what reason can be given why the configuration should have had any reference to it at all, or why the animal should not have gone on executing any one of an indefinite number of other movements which had no bearing upon the attainment of the goal ?

Once the point is admitted certain conclusions follow. The insight of the animal lay not in framing a continuous or a coherent set of movements, but in framing such a set as would lead to his attainment of his object. But, yet again, it was not the performance itself that constituted the intelligence, but the mental process that immediately preceded it. The new performance can be interpreted only as the objective outcome of the subjective occurrence.

We have, of course, abundant parallels to this on the higher level of human behaviour in corresponding circumstances. But if other evidence is required it is supplied by three phenomena which repeatedly accompanied the apes' solution. The first of these is the contemplative pause that preceded the act of insight. The second is the suddenness with which the successful performance was entered upon ; and the character of the performance, as of a new continuous whole, was the third. Leaving the first without comment, it is enough to point out that one cannot carry through with any confidence or suddenness, a new performance in its successive parts successfully, unless that performance is already " in one's head." If the solution had not dawned upon the ape, how could he possibly have proceeded to a fresh series of movements, so constructed and so ordered as to bring him and the object of his desire together, and have executed them with such little hesitation ? And can anyone reasonably maintain that after a series of unsuccessful performances, it is within the scope of probability that a consecutive chain of items different from those of the previous performances should have rolled itself off, yet just of the kind and order that the desired achievement demanded, except on the assumption that the animal possessed in a measure the power of apprehending the interrelations of these items beforehand in their bearing on the end desired ? The alternative to the hypothesis of a happy conglomeration of successful items lies not in an equally accidental configuration, but in this very capacity for becoming prospectively aware of the parts of a performance—a series of movements—relevant to the final or intended situation, in other words of the practical means to the end ; so that the animal can then act upon that insight. The subjective, in fine, conditions the objective. In what other terms can the performance be envisaged ? Yet a number of apes on several occasions achieved these consecutive new performances.

Two conclusions about the nature of the intelligence displayed in the apes' adjustment to the novel situations are therefore the following. One is that the act of intelligence was a mental process preceding the overt act ; the other that that process consisted, not in ' configuring ' as such, but in discovering, apprehending, or becoming aware of, a particular set of relations, namely the relations of a certain set of movements to one another in a whole performance, and the relation of the whole performance, or of the final movement of that performance, to the actual securing of the object. It was these relations that dawned upon the animal's mind.

On these considerations may now be based a provisional hypothesis of intelligence—intelligence as a capacity of the individual is a capacity to effect sub-jectively (that is, to apprehend), relevant relations and interrelations. By relevant is meant bearing on, and in their bearing on, some end or intended situation.

On this view the appropriateness of the ' configuration ' metaphor disappears. For the configuration does not exist in its own rights. The result of apprehending (and accommodating behaviour to) a succession of related movements and of apprehending these as related to a given end is that they will "fall into shape" or constitute a configuration. The configuration is not the explanation of the intelligent process, but is explained by it. The Gestalt psychologist puts the cart before the horse.

Of the propositions regarding intelligence, to be elaborated in the chapters that follow, it is convenient at this point to present the following :

1. Intelligence, as a distinctive psychological category, is a faculty or capacity to apprehend true or useful relations, or to discover subjectively, between objects, relations (using the word in the widest possible sense) that hold objectively.

2. This faculty is innate in the organism, and individuals differ from one another in the degree in which they possess the power. They are thus more, or less, intelligent.

3. The faculty functions at all levels on the evolutionary scale of life, but has reached its highest development in man. The same principle however obtains all along.

Since it is our contention that human individual mental development depends upon the exercise of intelligence rather than upon mechanical response to stimulus, we may devote the remainder of this chapter to a general consideration of intelligence in relation to learning, interpreting the term learning sufficiently liberally to include cognitive development generally.

Intelligence and the Learning Process

Before applying the present hypothesis of the psychological nature of intelligence to the problem of human learning it is as well to clear the ground by distinguishing two widely different uses of the *term* intelligence, which have hitherto served to obscure the issue. Suppose two men are making a comparative evaluation of a certain residence. Their valuations are found to differ widely. Discussion shows that while one has been thinking only of the house itself, the other had been including in his valuation the garden and grounds attached.

Similarly with intelligence we must first be clear what the *word* is intended to cover before we discuss the

nature of the thing we intend by it. In discussions on
the nature of intelligence discrepant uses of the *word*
(as distinct from the thing) often go unnoticed, and yet
(indeed for that very reason) cloud the argument ; for
it is where our implicit premises, held subconsciously,
differ that controversy becomes most hopeless, simply
because we remain unaware of the real grounds of our
disagreement.

Some people, considering the term intelligence, seem
to be intending at the back of their minds, the sum of
mental processes that make for efficiency. " What
is it," is their implicit question, " that makes A mentally
a more efficient person than B ? "

When this is the question at issue, the answer is of
course a comprehensive one. For clearly there is no
mental function excellence in which does not contribute
to general mental efficiency. A good power of recall,
vivid and exact imagination, sensory acuteness, facility
in attention, keenness of discrimination, and so on
(according to the particular classification of mental
functions favoured) all contribute their share to a
composite of general mental efficiency for the purposes
of life.

In contrast with this is the assumption that what we
have to seek is some particular function of the mind
which constitutes or involves intelligence, and stands
out or apart from the common list of functions, or
perhaps underlies or supports or serves them all.

On the first assumption intelligence is identified with
nothing *in particular*—it is a conglomerate of particular
abilities ;—on the second we arrive at some such doctrine,
say, as that it is the power of conceptual thinking, or of
attention, or of seizing the point of a question, and so on.
It is therefore important to insist that this present
discussion of intelligence suggests the conclusion that
a particular mental function does exist, hitherto most
inadequately recognized, which deserves the name of
intelligence par excellence ; and that on the recognition

of this faculty (the term faculty is not to be eschewed), a reform of our whole theory of cognition depends ; but that on the other hand it is equally true that other functions besides intelligence, as thus conceived, do contribute to general mental efficiency, and that therefore those who prefer to widen the connotation of the term to include all that makes for mental efficiency in life are of course at liberty to reject the limitations of the term as here proposed.

Those however who prefer this alternative must be prepared to discredit statements of the type " A is intelligent enough, but has a bad memory," or, Aristotle's claim " that a man's intelligence may be in inverse proportion to his memory," or " You are intelligent but you are inattentive," or " Helen Keller, though blind and dumb, is unusually intelligent." They would appear therefore to have popular usage against them. And if in the progress of our discussion it appears that intelligence in the sense now assigned to it, largely conditions the efficiency of the mind in all its aspects, and therefore mental efficiency in general, it will perhaps be conceded that its more serviceable connotation is the one now suggested.

However this may be, the reasons for drawing this distinction at this point are firstly, to forestall a possible confusion in the mind of the reader, and secondly to indicate that the interest of the present writer lies more in elucidating the character and significance of a faculty of cardinal psychological importance than in determining the question of its name.

On the other hand it is in place to add that for all psychologists who represent intelligence as the acquiring power, or adjustment to new situations, or the power to learn, or in similar terms, it is the psychological process which underlies those concepts which is being here considered.

The question now to be considered is of the application of intelligence in the sense given to the process of learning, that is, to the cognitive development of the individual through the use of his experience. For broadly speaking all successful adjustment to, or mastery of, new situations involves learning in the sense of acquisition of new skill or attainment of fresh knowledge.

In the case of animal learning experiments it is, of course, the latter, or intellectual, type of learning that has been usually, if not always, demanded. Of an ape in piling boxes, or of a rat threading a maze, no unfamiliar muscular co-ordinations are required in the movements which they execute. There is no new skill to be acquired. Human learning, however, exhibits a wide variety and range. There is the child learning to tie a knot, or lace up his shoes, or to sharpen a lead pencil without breaking the point, to solve mechanical puzzles (a problem most nearly akin to those set to Thorndike's cats) ; the burglar learning to break open a safe, or the prisoner to effect his escape from prison (a problem corresponding perhaps on the human plane, to those set by Köhler to his apes) ; there is learning to type or to play the piano, the youth learning baseball or tennis ; learning history, mathematics, or psychology ; the author composing a story ; the painter creating a picture ; the poet his poem ; Napoleon planning a campaign ; Newton discovering the law of gravitation ; and Shakespeare creating Hamlet.

For the purpose of disclosing intelligence at work in meeting novel situations all these are instances of learning, just as are the minor adaptations of daily domestic demands, as in following a new recipe, dealing with a refractory child, scrubbing a new room, or coping with any of the indefinite number of petty problems that arise every day and hour, and almost every minute, of our daily lives.

Though it is no doubt convenient to select certain striking cases of rather elaborate new acquisitions for purposes of demonstrative analysis, this need not obscure the fact that learning is a constant process in human life, and that the same psychological principle of intelligence is at work all along ; and that the learning process in every case exhibits certain constant common features.

Of these two are cardinal to our discussion, namely, repetition and variation ; identity and difference. Take the case of the small boy learning to sharpen his pencil with a pocket knife. His process of acquiring this petty skill illustrates the co-operation of these two factors ; he has used his knife for general purposes already, and has learnt to cut pieces of wood with it. He now attempts for the first time to sharpen a pencil. The process of acquiring skill begins with rather rough and clumsy strokes at the pencil end, with slices too deep and disproportionate, and he frequently breaks the lead point by too heavy a pressure. With practice however his strokes gain in delicacy, his pressure becomes more even and the shape more symmetrical and the pencil point sharper. Each stage in the achievement is marked by repetitions of previously acquired co-ordinations, with slight modifications or variations of them in the direction desired.

There is a constant succession of repetitions with variations, and of repetitions *of variations*, or of the previous movements more or less modified. The progress, the essential learning, consists not in the repetitions but in the variations ; and in further variations as each previous variation is established. It is not the identities that constitute the learning pattern so much as the differences.

This fact must be faced by those psychologists who maintain that learning is only a reinstatement of past experience, or a selection from amongst activities previously acquired or inherited. The reverse of this appears to be the truth. It is in newness of performance that the learning—the progress—depends. Not that repetition, or previous experience, is superfluous. On the contrary it is essential to the learning. Every new achievement leans upon, and embodies, the old. There is no such thing as a completely new creation. And every new performance, every variation or innovation must become old in its turn, before fresh innovations can be built upon it. Conservation conditions creation, consolidation conditions advance.

But now let us ask where, even in so humble a skill, the factor of intelligence comes in. From his first attempts to sharpen the pencil properly the motions of the boy's fingers are never random. He has, and is aware of, a definite end. His very first movements are undertaken with intelligence ; intelligence of a low degree, certainly, well within the reach of every normal being, and of animals as well ; but still intelligence. He could not have made his pencil sharp without it. For his very initial strokes imply that he has already apprehended the relation of the movement to the object in view ; else he could not have made the movement ; unless we assume—and surely no one will seriously assume—that the growing boy has an instinctive impulse for sharpening lead pencils, and that his performance-series or detailed process of sharpening them is innately determined apart from experience.

And in selecting each useful variation which is in turn established, some degree of intelligence is also at work. He apprehends for example that the better point, or the more symmetrical shape, is related to the lighter pressure, else why should he persevere with it, why repeat and confirm it, rather than a heavier pressure or a different kind of stroke ?

And here a point of some interest comes in. It is not necessary for this apprehension of relations, for the consciousness of the relation to be either intense or explicit. Mental process—serving as it does life's practical purposes—is marked throughout by a convenient economy of consciousness. In the rapid play of movement which takes place in the sharpening of a pencil, no high degree of awareness is necessary for apprehending, and immediately acting upon, a perceptual relation of the movement to the end. Had the operator been a professor of psychology, whose purpose was to explain afterwards to his class his mental processes in learning to sharpen the pencil, the case would have been otherwise. He would actively have attended to what was going on. He would, that is, have thus raised to a higher level of clearness the awareness of the fact that the delicate stroke meant the sharper point or the better shape, for he would have needed to recall it, and attention facilitates recall. Moreover his consciousness would have been explicit : that is, so clearly defined and determinate, as to be expressible in words ; it would have reached the level of verbal awareness. But for the boy's immediate purpose neither of these achievements was required. He had neither to recall the relations on both occasions, nor to communicate his experience to others. For his immediate purpose—and that is all he was concerned with at the time—the dimmest and most fleeting apprehension sufficed, just enough to pass over to his immediately following movements. Hence there can be no wonder that if the boy were asked afterwards whether he saw at the time the relation on which he based his action he would have recalled no such awareness.

The universality of this economy of consciousness constitutes it not a mere fact but a psychological law. Its biological import is obvious. To be conscious as the necessities of the situations demand has obvious survival value : to be more conscious than the situations demand, or to be burdened with consciousness of other things, is to waste mental energy, and to court mental confusion.

It is thus an instance of " the happy economy of nature " that in cases of motor learning intelligence acts or functions almost unaware. There is no need for impressed awareness, for the new muscular co-ordinations are establishing themselves with practice, and save the need of explicit recall. On the next occasion *they* repeat the performance : there is no need to recall it. Contrast with this the case of intellectual learning. To learn a poem one must be clearly conscious of the words. It is them one has to recall. To solve a mechanical puzzle one must be clearly aware of the principles involved in the solution if one is to be sure of solving it aright next time ; one must, that is to say, have made explicit to oneself the relations one has apprehended, for they are to be recalled when the situation recurs.

The law is nicely exemplified in cases where one acquires a skill by first apprehending the principles which the acquisition entails, as in learning to steer a bicycle, or to type. In mastering a bicycle one bears in mind with almost painful intensity the actual relations involved in accurate steering ; but after a month's riding, when the muscular co-ordinations are set, the relations have almost slipped out of mind, and a time is eventually reached when it requires an effort of memory to be able to communicate them to another learner.

This law of economy of consciousness has been dwelt upon, because its bearing upon the process of intelligence awaits adequate recognition. The possible objection is forestalled, that because there has been no easily recallable consciousness of the relations apprehended, therefore intelligence has been absent in the acquisition. The answer to this objection is that it would be strange indeed—and would require special explanation—if a law, whose application is generally recognized in the class of case just mentioned, should be found to cease to apply in other cases when the conditions for its functioning were the same. But the case of intelligent apprehensions should be no exception to the rule.[1]

For our second example of learning can be taken the processes involved in mastering a game, say tennis. As in the case of sharpening the pencil, there is of course, involved an improvement, with practice, in the delicacy and exactness of muscular co-ordination. Over the details of these the player has no conscious control. But he has control over the gross movements, which require them. He selects and directs these movements. His early efforts are directed to getting the ball over the net, so as to fall within the limits of the opposite court. Intelligent activity, the apprehension, for example, of the relation of a certain strength of stroke to the place where the ball will drop, of a certain angle of the racquet to the course which the ball will follow in the air, of a certain position of his body to that of the ball and of this relation to ease of returning the ball, and so on, is involved here, just as in the sharpening of the pencil. Such intelligent activity is within the range of every ordinary person.

It may be noted, however, that here again each improvement in skill entails repetition and variation, and it is the variation that is the condition of all progress. As and when the player apprehends the relation of a certain strength of stroke to a position in the middle of the opposite court, his previous movements (running towards the ball, swinging his right arm to meet it, etc.) repeat themselves, but with a modification—a change, say, in the speed of the meeting movement. And this change, after apprehending its relation to the drop of the ball within the limits desired, he proceeds to reiterate and confirm. And increasing skill in the game is dependent on a succession of fresh relational achievements, the apprehension, for example, of the relation of a shot down the side line to the constancy of position of an opponent, and of his body and his " back hand " to the spot where such a shot will fall ; of the relation of a certain style of service stroke to the angle at which the ball bounces, and of this again to the actual or customary receiving position of the opponent ; or the apprehension again of a whole number of relations between the observed weak points of an opponent to certain types of stroke or certain tactics of the player himself.

Achieving skill in the game involves a succession of apprehensions of relationships, each built up on, and succeeding, a fundamental system of relationships already established ; and as each new point in the game is ' seized,' acted on, and " made one's own," so the mind is set free to seize upon new ones, a prelude to further progress.

Other things being equal (important among them being zeal and physical capacity) the more intelligent player will apprehend these relations more readily, and in the later stages apprehend more complex relations, and will keep on increasing his advance upon his duller competitor at every stage.

That it is the variations or the differences that constitute the essence of the learning is, of course, still more evident in the case of intellectual learning ; in which the new acquisition is that of a fact or principle, and no practice in motor co-ordinations appears, at first sight at least, to be necessary for progress, or for adjustment to novel conditions.   Instances of intellectual learning might be taken, the solution of a mechanical puzzle, a scientific discovery,and—to go to the school curriculum— the learning of history.   In each of these cases the learning depends on (if indeed it does not consist in) the direct apprehension of a relation, or the functioning of intelligence.

The process of solving mechanical puzzles is particularly pertinent, because it exemplifies, in a certain sense, the adoption of methods of trial-and-error as a means towards solution, and might seem at first sight, to support the trial-and-error doctrine of learning.   Thus Ruger's[2] subjects, presented with a number of toy mechanical puzzles, often resorted to random movements of different parts of the mechanisms on the chance of some of the resulting changes of position either clarifying the situation or actually constituting the solution (or part of it).   Just similarly have all of us, I suppose, in disentangling a tangle of string, pulled threads of it at random here and there, and thus frequently successfully unravelled it.

But it must be carefully noted that the adoption of a method of trial-and-error in cases like these differs from the process of trial-and-error as conceived by advocates of a mechanistic explanation of learning in one crucial respect, namely, in the presence of intelligence behind it.   When we resort to trial-and-error in unravelling a tangle of string we do so because we are aware that the string is in such a tangle that the apprehension of its various important spatial relations would take more time and trouble than a disentanglement by random pulls and tugs.   In other words we intelligently adopt an ' unintelligent ' method.   This contrasts, in the one crucial point—the presence of a directing intelligence—with the (assumed) random trials of Thorndike's cats, or of rats in a maze.   For precisely the same reason an intelligent human being will adopt trial-and-error methods in solving toy puzzles.   He knows that they are cleverly contrived to conceal the significant relationships, while at the same time their limited number of parts and their comparatively simple structure offer a good chance of success by rapidly trying a variety of random moves.   It is thus the more significant that even in a case like this, where the conditions are selectively set to favour trial-and-error methods, the dependence of the solution of the puzzles upon the capacity to apprehend relations is abundantly illustrated.

Ruger's experiment is the more interesting in that it exemplifies this act of apprehension as it occurs at different levels of consciousness, from the low level remarked in the boy learning to sharpen a pencil, to the sudden flash or dawn of an idea witnessed again and again in Köhler's apes.   Speaking of the way in which variations or innovations were introduced " At one extreme," writes Ruger, " is the motor variation which perhaps brings success, but which runs its course unnoticed. At the other extreme the analysis (that is, our awareness of particular relations) may come first and only after a considerable interval be followed by the motor response. Or again, simultaneous but distinguished—a flash of insight and a motor response. Or one may notice later the significance of a movement unconsciously (that is, unwittingly) begun. The technique of the acquisition of skill in manipulation is in these humble cases in accord with the complex thinking processes, viz. a variation set up as a hypothesis, tested and accepted for control purposes or rejected as the case may be."[3] Of the sudden insight sometimes experienced Ruger says, " It is oftentimes a striking experience, and seems to come with a rush or as a flash. Sometimes the subject seemed to see the relations involved in the solution directly, and without the use of imagery."[4]

But it is not, of course, to be supposed that the variations on first occurrence were always the result of a previous act of apprehension—in conditions so favourable for the deliberate practice of trial methods the variations would constantly take the form of random moves. Intelligence would then appear in apprehending the true (or useful) bearing of the variation on the end in view after the variation had been tried, since it is much easier to detect relations between elements presented in the concrete than if they are merely thought of. On the other hand to be able to dispense with the concrete is one index of a superior intelligence.

It is also significant—a point again observed in Ruger's experiments—that the apprehension of a variation or fresh relation does not necessarily

(1) affect practice immediately afterwards, nor

(2) having affected it, inevitably recur on the next occasion. In fact, it may never recur at all.

The reasons for these delays or vacillations are not

hard to seek. One may apprehend a relation, but yet not at the time also apprehend the relation of that relation to the end in view, for it is frequently a relational complex that has to be apprehended. Later on, when the situation recurs the previous relation is reinstated, more determinately, and therefore more securely, and one is in a position to apprehend its place in the solution also. Or again, one may entertain in succession two or more hypotheses (assumed relationships) and one of these may escape memory while another is being tried out.

That a hypothesis or solution is not always repeated on the next occasion is still more easily accounted for as an ordinary case of failure to recall. Probably few of us but have experienced the annoyance of forgetting some solution of a problem (say, a mathematical problem) or of some plan or project conceived by us a short time previously.

Even Thorndike's cats were not exempt from a similar weakness ; the recurrence of a situation by no means always reinstates the solution previously successful. Thorndike cites this as a sign of absence of intelligence.[5] The reverse is rather the explanation. For if the creature were mechanical, though subject also—as Thorndike supposes—to the " stamping in " effect of pleasure—the reinstatement of the situation would inevitably and invariably have occasioned the previous reaction. For memory and intelligence are, by his hypothesis, excluded. But the lapse is intelligible enough if we assume either that the creatures had grasped the solution but forgot it (human beings even forget, and surely lower animals no less), or, as is equally possible, had as suggested above, so far inadequately grasped a relational complex.

We may now turn, for our last illustration, to a kind of learning of which the essential akinness in principle to those already mentioned requires to be recognized, namely, creative imagination. A single brief instance

may for the moment suffice.   A poetical simile.   Wrote
the poet Shelley,

> " Life, like a dome of many-coloured glass,
> Stains the white radiance of eternity,
> Until death tramples it to fragments."

The reader is struck by the beauty of the comparison.
What precisely constitutes its beauty is not, however,
the point here at issue, but it can at least be claimed
that it could not have been beautiful if it had not first
been appropriate.   But in what does its appropriateness
consist ?   In relationships between the two experiences
compared, and in nothing else.   Once the poet has
pointed out these relationships, we admit them readily
enough.   The wonderful variety, the intensity, the
brightness of life, and the unfathomability, the mystery
of the encompassing eternity into which at a stroke it
vanishes, each of these aspects is clearly exhibited by
the simile.   To effect such a simile whole sets of relations
must have dawned or flashed upon the mind of the poet.
And where we marvel at his achievement most is in his
power of selecting out of a host of possible objects of
comparison, one which offered so many relationships
to the main concept, life, in so graphic and simple a form.
There   perhaps   lay   Shelley's   super-intelligence,   his
genius.

So with the scientific imagination of a Newton, a
Darwin, or an Einstein.   It consists in an unusual
capacity to apprehend relations and relational systems
more comprehensive, more far-reaching, more fundamental, than the ordinary individual is capable of.
This is aptitude for the highest work in science, as in
poetry, or any occupation ; for all work truly original
depends upon just this capacity—on unusual intelligence,
that is, the power of ' seeing ' more than others see ;
for seeing ahead of one's fellows.   Such are " men of
vision," the intellectual leaders of men.

Our hypothesis of intelligence thus far provisionally advanced may now be clarified and checked by an examination of the two contrasted views of this faculty held by Thorndike and by Spearman respectively. To this are devoted the next two chapters.

CHAPTER VI

THORNDIKE ON INTELLIGENCE

I. *The Nature of Intelligence*

PROFESSOR THORNDIKE, so far at least as his theoretical principles are concerned, is a leading exponent of the reaction-hypothesis or 'stimulus-response' school of psychology. Now as has been pointed out[1] according to the strict logic of this school there is no place available in human behaviour for intelligence as such, that is for any distinctive power or faculty of intelligence apart from the automatic response of the organism to environmental stimuli ; and all that can consistently be conveyed by the term intelligence is a high proportion of 'successful' responses (whatever be our criterion of success), remembering that the successes are the outcome of the stimuli on the one hand and of the individual's particular set of innate reaction-patterns on the other.

Thorndike himself, more consistently with this position than some of the mechanistic school, describes intelligence as the power of good responses from the point of view of truth or fact. Not wholly consistently however, for though the word responses is appropriate, a sensory stimulus acting on a sense organ has itself no knowledge of truth or fact and so no power of selecting its responses according to truth or fact ; so that either the correspondence with truth or fact is accidental, in which case the word *power* is out of place, or if we retain the word 'power', then there is introduced some additional capacity of or in the organism to judge truth or fact, other than the automatic reactions of the human mechanism to its environment

58

However that may be, a general description of this sort is of little psychological value, for it tells us nothing of the mental processes concerned in producing the good responses and does not explain what is meant by good or bad responses.

More in keeping with his general position was Thorndike's former contention that intelligence consists of a multiplicity of innate abilities, a " compound of many traits ",[2] the mind being a " multitude of functions each of which involves content as well as form and so is closely related to only a few of its fellows, to the others with greater and greater degrees of remoteness."[3] In the same spirit he says, " Good reasoning power is only the name for a host of particular capacities and incapacities, the general average of which seems to the namer to be above the average in other individuals."[4] This view of a multiplicity of factors was held in opposition to the view which Thorndike has explicitly criticised " that all branches of intellectual activity are bound to each other in all cases by one common factor."[5] On the other hand Thorndike also asserts that all branches of intellectual activity " are positively correlated."[6] In fine he has hitherto maintained (1) that ' intelligent ' reactions are so many separate responses to situations or stimuli, and (2) that they nevertheless are positively correlated. The difficulty arises of accounting for the correlation.

In his recent publication entitled *The Measurement of Intelligence* we have a chapter devoted to " The Nature of Intellect " which attacks this problem. The remarkably close correlation which intelligence tests have evidenced between different expressions or overt products of intelligence cannot be satisfactorily accounted for by mere coincidences or by the chance occurrence of high averages. Thorndike is therefore in search of a unitary factor. " One cherishes the hope that some simpler, more unitary fact exists as the cause of intellect and that variations in the magnitude of this fact may provide a single fundamental scale which will account for levels

and range and surface."[7]   This means that the existence
of some general factor, some general ability, is now
recognized by Thorndike, in which individuals differ and
which accounts for the differences. The tenor of the
book as a whole testifies to this change of attitude.
" Presumably a man can use intellect and display the
amount of it which he possesses in operations with any
sort of material object, any living plant or animal,
including himself, any quality or relation that exists
in reality or in imagination, any idea or emotion or
act."[8] Provisionally intellect is defined as "that
quality of mind (or brain or behaviour if one prefers)
in respect to which Aristotle, Plato, Thucydides, and
the like, differed most from Athenian idiots of their
day, or in respect to which lawyers, physicians, scientists,
scholars, and editors of reputed greatest ability at
constant age, say a dozen of each, differ most from idiots
of that age in our asylums."[9] " We have assumed that
(1) there is such a quality or characteristic of man as
altitude or level of intellect ; (2) whose amount or
degree is measured by the height at which it can attain
success with a series of intellectual tasks ranked for
difficulty."[10] " In the case of intellect it is well worth
while to seek rigorous measures of intellectual difficulty,
because intellect is so important an ability and because
altitude of intellect turns out to be a fairly unified,
coherent variable properly represented by cardinal
numbers,"[11] and so on. This is the language of a
multiple theory of intelligence no longer.

But the difficulty remains of reconciling this acceptance of a general fact or ability with the requirements
of the reaction-hypothesis or association psychology.
It is this reconciliation we have now to examine.

To help in the solution of the problem recourse is
had to specially undertaken experiments, comparisons
being made of the performances of a number of school
students of different school grades in selected so-called
purely associative and higher processes respectively.

" As measures of the ' higher ' or ' control ' abilities he (the experimenter) used sentence completions, arithmetical problems, and analogies tests. As measures of the purely ' associative ' abilities he used vocabulary tests, routine and informational arithmetic, and information tests."[12]   On the basis of these Thorndike arrives at certain conclusions of importance :

(1) That the higher mental abilities are the same in kind as the lower level or purely associative processes ;

(2) That the kind in which they are the same is mere association, and the higher processes involve in the main no cognitive process other than association ;

(3) That the difference between a greater and a lesser degree of native intelligence is a difference in the number, not in the kind, of associations of which the individual is capable.

These conclusions derive from the test results in the following fashion. Comparing the tests of students in higher or control abilities and purely ' associative ' abilities respectively, correlations result of which the following are typical :

Higher with higher .53

Lower with lower .64$\frac{1}{5}$

Higher with lower .57

What is common to two higher with what is common to two lower .94.

" These facts," runs the argument, " are almost crucial. They prove that mere association and the higher abilities have in the main the same cause.   Almost all of whatever is common to the one sort is common to the other sort." This establishes proposition (1).

This however would not of itself seem sufficient to establish proposition (2).   One would naturally argue that since the cause was common one is entitled to seek for it just as much in the higher as in the lower abilities. It might be that by examining intelligence where it functions at its highest level, where, that is, it is most intelligent, we should find the common factor which also appears at the lower level. This notion however is rejected by Thorndike as absurd. " If we are to avoid the conclusion," he writes, " that associative ability is this cause, we must either place the causation of associative ability in the higher ability, or seek a common cause for both which is different from either, such as a general mental energy or vitality. The first of these assumptions is absurd, because associative ability occurs abundantly without any trace of the higher abilities, but these never occur without it. In the lower animals, in idiots, and low imbeciles, and in the young infant, mental connections are formed without the appearance or use of abstraction, generalization or relational thinking."[15] This is held to establish proposition (2).

The argument is ingenious, but it requires something other than intelligence to be able to detect the particular absurdity referred to. That there is something common to the two sets of mental processes is a fair conclusion, but the statistical results which Thorndike gives are not specially favourable to his argument. That the common element in the lower processes correlates highly with the common element in the higher processes merely indicates that an element present in doing the ' associative ' exercises is also present in doing the more intellectually exacting exercises, and if that common element is intelligence or the cause of intelligence (as Thorndike maintains) it is perfectly consistent with the view that an ability pre-eminent in the higher processes is also in some measure present in the lower. This common factor and not mere associative ability as such is what the statistical statement equally admits as the common cause.

So far, then, as Thorndike's statistical *ad hoc* evidence goes, it is equally compatible with either interpretation, that intelligent process is purely associative, or that the " associative processes " used in the experiments are not the purely associative affairs he claims they are.

But it should be noted that the plausibility of Thorndike's argument depends on begging the question at issue. He begins by assuming that vocabulary tests, routine and informational arithmetic and information tests involve purely associative processes. He begins, that is to say, by assuming the very thing he is out to prove, namely that mental operations are purely associative, and that the particular exercises he has selected to test this very point are purely associative operations. If indeed the so-called " purely associative " processes are what they are assumed to be then the proposition that the higher abilities and mere association have in the main the same cause and have the same derivation is at least consistent with his premise, but even so it does not follow that the higher processes are merely associative. For, admit that the higher processes are derived from the associative abilities, we have yet no more right to claim on that ground that they are both mere association than we have to claim that because oak trees are derived from acorns oak trees and acorns are the same things. We know they are not.

Having, however, concluded that associative ability is the cause of intelligence, Thorndike faces the question what meaning can we attach to the terms higher and lower degrees of intelligence. What is meant by saying that A is more intelligent than B ? Can we represent the difference between the capacity for the higher and that for the lower processes in psychological terms ? An answer to this question in terms of *quality* of intellectual process has already been ruled out, for as we have seen the cardinal process for both the more and the less intelligent activities is assumed to be association. But an answer is forthcoming in terms of quantity. " The hypothesis which we shall present and shall defend," writes Thorndike, " admits the distinction (namely distinction of quality) in respect of surface behaviour, but asserts that in their deeper nature the higher forms of intellectual operation are identical with

mere association or connection forming, depending upon
the same sort of physiological connections but requiring
*many more of them.** By the same argument the person
whose intellect is greater or higher or better than that
of another person differs from him in the last analysis
in having, not a new sort of physiological process, but
simply a larger number of connections of the ordinary
sort."[16] Intelligence then is higher or lower according
to the number of connections of which the individual
is capable, to his original capacity for a larger number
of connections. " The original possibility of having
more such connections "[17] which is the cause of the
original differences in intellect among men, is for
convenience symbolized by a big C, a little c standing
for the possibility of one connection.[18] " What is
essential to the hypothesis is that by original nature,
men differ in respect of the number of connections or
associations with ideas which they can form, so that
despite identical outside environments, some of them
would have many more than others." " Negatively
the hypothesis asserts that no special qualitative
differences are required to account for differences in
degree of intellect ; the higher processes or powers
have no other basis in original nature than that which
accounts for differences in the number of bonds of the
associative type."[19]

' C ' then, the " Physiological parallel of number of
mental connections "[20] is assumed to be the fact that
underlies ability in the higher as in the lower processes.
The difference between the greater and lesser intelligence
is one purely of number of associations of which the
individual is capable.

But let us consider the implications of the hypothesis
that the difference between the higher and the lower
intelligence consists in the power of the one to form
more connections than the other. Now Thorndike has
already pointed out, indeed it is vital to his theory,

*The italics are Thorndike's.

that associative ability occurs abundantly in idiots and imbeciles ; and he selects purely associative processes as characteristic of the low type of intelligence. To think on the purely associative level and to be unintelligent are by his hypothesis synonymous. And no doubt the ordinary intelligent person will have little difficulty in according agreement : he will agree that the stupidities of the unintelligent are just of this nature—they seem to be purely associative processes. Take for instance a simple instance of the Analogies test : " complete with the fitting word from those given : Prisoner is to jail as water is to Prison, Drink, Tap, Bucket." We find the unintelligent person stupidly selecting ' drink,' the intelligent person ' bucket ' as the completion of the analogy. And the reason is clear. ' Drink ' has been previously experienced *in association* with ' water ' —hence this word recurs irrespective of its actual appropriateness. The stupidity is obvious. It consists in the functioning of a " purely associative " process. Whereas the intelligent person sees the greater *appropriateness* of ' bucket '. But surely no one can really be expected to accept Thorndike's hypothesis that the cardinal difference between the unintelligent and the intelligent person lies in the greater number of stupidities of which the intelligent person is capable, that he has a greater capacity for making stupid mistakes.

It was perhaps suspicion of the absurdity to which his hypothesis committed him that induced Thorndike to conclude his discussion of the theory of intelligence with a significant qualification. After satisfying himself that ' C ' is the *main* cause of intellect or the higher abilities, and dismissing the alternative assumption that the cause may be discerned in the higher abilities themselves, he introduces quite a number of qualifying factors. " We do not maintain that C is the sole cause of intellect in original nature, so that two persons with identical numbers of C's and identical training will necessarily have identical intellectual achievements."

Amongst these other factors " there is also perhaps ", we read, " a capacity for having the neurones *act with reference one to another*,* that is, with *integration*, whose low or negative extreme is pronounced dissociation as in hysteria, and whose higher positive extreme appears as a notable good sense or adequacy in the use of one's experiences.   This capacity maybe is largely irrespective of C."[21]

This seems to be a belated admission, though stated in more than questionable physiological terms, of a part played in intelligent activity by relevant or consistent thinking, and that the causative factor of intelligence may after all be found in this conspicuous characteristic of the higher abilities.   Thus what he has rejected as absurd on one page he appears to welcome back on the page following.   But in so doing he has cut away the foundations of his whole psychological system.   Its prime principle of behaviour is mechanical response to stimulus.   But to endow your neurones with a mysterious power of acting in reference one to another, and to admit that human intelligent behaviour is partly determined by their doing so, is no longer to hold that human behaviour can be adequately rendered in terms of mechanical response to stimuli, or human mental processes in terms of pure association.

It is much to be deplored that Thorndike should have devoted only one or two sentences in one short paragraph in his book to this important reservation.   The serious student of psychology is naturally anxious to know what precisely is denoted by the " capacity for having the neurones act *with reference one to another, that is, with* integration."   Is it intended to imply that each neurone has some power in itself of considering the wants and desires of its brother neurones, or is it only a physiological metaphor to indicate the power of the individual mind to apprehend relevancies or to integrate its experiences ? If the former, whence does Thorndike get his evidence

*The italics are Thorndike's.

that the neurones have these independent personalities ?
If the latter, why use the misleading 'neuronic'
phraseology at all ? The curious and presumably
considered use of the phrase "having the neurones"
do so-and-so seems to imply the interpolation of
individual volition, or of some control over the neurones
by the individual as an individual. So important a
thesis deserves elaboration.

II. *Is Intelligence Mere Association ?*

The inconsistencies which invalidate Thorndike's
arguments about intelligence seem to have derived
historically from his early espousal of one radically
extreme position in opposition to another.

It will be remembered that more than a quarter of a
century ago Thorndike was a leader in an attack, fully
justified no doubt at the time, against an extreme and
uncritically anthropomorphic view of the nature of
animal intelligence. He confronted the enemy with the
weapons of experiment and of an associationist and
physiological psychology. And although, no doubt
largely through his lead, the danger he scented has
passed away, there is nothing like success for concealing
and confirming the weaknesses of one's own position.

So far as the present discussion is concerned, the
root fallacy lies in confusing two meanings of the
term 'association', or—more exactly—in recognizing
'association' in one of its senses, the sense consonant
with the 'ism' in question, while ignoring it in the
other.

It is of course true that in all 'intelligent' process
objects of consciousness do occur together, and in this
sense all thinking entails association. I cannot, for
instance, complete the analogy mentioned in the previous
section without being conscious of 'prisoner' and
'water' and 'drink' and 'bucket', etc. That objects
may occur together in consciousness is one of the
conditions of thinking. But what the 'pure association'

theory of Thorndike and his followers persistently overlooks is that thinking, intelligent process, does not consist in the mere association, the juxtaposition in consciousness, of objects or ideas.

To make clear this point and to illustrate the difference between the two kinds of association does not require experimental evidence. For there is clearly another sense in which I may be said to 'associate' ideas. There is present to my consciousness, to take an instance, or I entertain the ideas of, the eating of raw strawberries and indigestion. Probably the reader, as he reads these words, has already experienced more than the mere having these two ideas together in consciousness. He has 'actively associated' in a particular way. He has thought of the eating of the strawberries as *causing* the indigestion. In other words he has effected or apprehended a particular kind of relation between two objects of thought. But this is not the only relation he may have apprehended between them. He may have cognized the strawberries as preventing the indigestion, or as preceding it, or even as having nothing to do with it, and so on. This kind of association, it will be noted, is an active mental affair, and the thinking is not just having the two ideas together in consciousness but relating the objects to which they refer in a very special and particular way. In fact it is not the objects of consciousness but the act of relating them that is the very essence of the thinking. It is, to put it crudely, the transitional process between the objects 'associated' (in the former sense of passive association) that is the distinctive mark of the thinking. To association in the latter sense of active, the awareness of one kind of relation rather than another subsisting between the objects of thought, the term 'relating' is probably the more appropriate ; and will serve to avoid the neglect of an element vital in thinking that comes of a needless linguistic confusion. It is just this power of relating objects of consciousness that is the characteristic of intelligent thought.

Now no amount of 'associating' or merely having two objects together in consciousness will account for this relating that takes place between them. All that association yields is the separate objects present simultaneously or in succession; but no amount of "having together" matches and flames in my mind will account for my establishing a particular relation between the two. The problem of *intelligence* in a word is not even touched by the "merely associative ability" hypothesis which Thorndike is compelled by his 'ism' to make his mainstay.

Having then no place for quality of mental process, the theory in keeping with its premises resorts to an explanation of superior intelligence in terms of quantity or number of associations. But on such a principle people like Miss Bates in Jane Austen's *Emma*, whose consciousness teemed with 'associations' would be on a higher intelligence level than a slower but more coherent thinker who might yet be a Darwin. And mere rapidity of succession of associations would be the mark of the superior intelligence. But while Miss Bates thought "in zig-zags" Darwin thought "to the point." How can mere number of associations account for this difference in quality?

On the theory of mere association a raving lunatic jabbering his multitude of incoherent and chaotic ideas may evidence an intelligence level superior to the sober student thinking steadily and relevantly to his subject.

That Thorndike saves himself from this absurdity only by a minor reservation in equivocal terms and disposed of in a single paragraph is a practical confession of the inadequacy of his main thesis, and at the same time of his inability to raise his reservation to the dignity of a leading principle because it is incompatible with his associationist doctrine.

In reply to this we shall perhaps be told, indeed we are told, that the capacity of thinking to the point is a matter of training.   " The hypothesis which we present," writes Thorndike, " . . . credits the quality of the ideas that a man acquires and the truth or falsity of the judgment which he makes, and to some extent even the validity of the inferences which he draws from any given data largely to his training."[22]   But, it may well be asked, how can we train a capacity which, by hypothesis, does not exist ?   And again why should we ?   If superior intelligence is only making more associations, all you need do in order to exercise your intelligence better is to train yourself to associate more abundantly.   Why should, and how could, quality ever come in ?   To admit the importance and the possibility of quality is to admit a capacity for quality (and not only quantity) already existing to be trained.   Thus Thorndike ends by contradicting in effect his own hypothesis.

III. *A Physiological Rendering of Intelligence*

Some comment is required on the use made by Thorndike and others of physiology in their account of intelligence and mental processes generally.   The physiological is one way of approach to psychological phenomena, but dangers beset the path of the investigator who sets out to study one science through the medium of another ;   particularly when as in the cases of psychology and physiology the phenomena of the two sciences are so different in kind as to be mutually irreducible.   For physiology is concerned with material and psychology primarily with immaterial happenings, neither adequately explicable in terms of the other.

The danger of the physiological approach is that of pre-occupying the student with the material aspect of his subject and of prejudicing him through that pre-occupation, nay more, of rendering him blind to more specifically psychical phenomena.   And when in addition he approaches his study with the assumption that all explanation is necessarily mechanistic (an assumption which will be examined in a later chapter) there is no only a danger, there is a certainty, that he will fail to view his subject in its own perspective.

A few citations from Thorndike's short chapter on the " Nature of Intellect " will indicate this ' physiological ' tendency. " One realizes the desirability of search for the physiological cause of intellect, regardless of whether that cause be single or simple or manifold and complex."[23] " The hypothesis which we present asserts that in their deeper nature the higher forms of intellectual operation are identical with mere association or connection forming, depending upon the same sort of physiological connections but requiring many more of them. By the same argument the person whose intellect is greater or higher or better than that of another person differs from him in the last analysis in having, not a new sort of physiological process, but simply a larger number of connections of the ordinary sort."[24] " Let c represent whatever anatomical or physiological fact corresponds to the possibility of forming one connection or association or bond between an idea or any part or aspect or feature thereof and a sequent idea or movement or any part or aspect or feature thereof."[25] Of the person of superior intelligence we read " his greater fund of ideas and connections is partly due to larger life and more varied and stimulating life, but it may be and certainly is partly due to original nature. It has some anatomical or physiological cause or parallel. Our hypothesis regards this anatomical cause or correspondence of the original possibility of having more such connections (call it C) as the causes of the original differences in intellect among men."[26] In addition to C, we read, intellect may entail a " capacity for having neurones act *with reference one to another,* that is, with *integration.*" Regarding the nature of C he writes " any person familiar with the finer anatomy of the brain will at once think of the number of possible contacts (or possible coalescences) of the fibrils of axones with dendritic processes in the associative neurones which act in perception, thought and speech as a highly probable C. We have it in mind as the possible C which we should investigate first if opportunity offered."[27]

There is of course much help derived in the study of psychological processes from making a parallel study of their physiological correspondents ; psychology owes a big debt to the physiological psychologist. But even if we admit—what is unproven—that every psychical process or event has its physiological correspondent, that does not warrant us in preferring for a psychical faculty or function a definition in physiological terms. To render intelligence in physiological language is no step towards a definition of it. Far less is it an explanation of it. One of the dangers of the resort to physiological descriptions and ' definitions ' of intelligence is that they produce the impression, and seem intended to produce the impression, that if we can only state the psychical process in ' bodily ' language we have somehow reduced the process to something more real, more adequate, less mysterious, and more satisfactory than it was in the original. It is indeed the ambition of the stimulus-response psychology which Thorndike professes, and which others have attempted to elaborate, to effect this very reduction. But why should this peculiar preference be accorded to the material over the immaterial ; in what sense if any is the former a more valid kind of experience ? There is no shred of evidence that a toothache is any less·real or less intelligible (though one may admit it is less satisfying) than a tooth, or the emotion of fright than the fire which occasioned it, or my love for a friend than is its object. There is nothing more real or intelligible or less mysterious about the latter class of phenomena. There is thus no reason " in the nature of things " for resort to the physiological rendering.

Moreover even if we admit a thorough psycho-physical parallelism and can hope to find a physiological parallel for every known psychical process, a knowledge of the physiological correspondent of a psychical phenomenon can do nothing whatever to elucidate the phenomenon as such. We cannot even begin to search for the physiological correspondent until we have the psychical process before us first. It is impossible to infer a psychical process from a physiological unless we are already familiar with the psychical process directly. The physiological can of itself give us no hint whatever as to the psychical process corresponding to it. No amount of physiological investigation can yield directly any psychical data.

Not even were we able to disclose all the intricate activities of the 900,000,000 nerve cells of the cerebral cortex should we be thereby a step advanced towards the knowledge of a single additional psychical fact. The facts can be obtained in one and only one way, by the direct revelation of our own consciousness. Having thus first ascertained them, we can then proceed to discover, if we can, what goes on in the nervous system or in the body more generally when one or other of those psychic events happen ; but this in no way helps us to know these events themselves. Therefore explanation of psychical phenomena in the sense of consistent coherent systematization under laws and principles, is necessarily a psychological and not a physiological process, and it can never consist in the reference of psychical events to physiological correspondents.

It is one danger then of the physiological treatment of psychology that it beguiles us with illusory physiological ' explanations.' A second is that of diverting us from the true quest. Excessive attention to the physiological aspects of one's subject reduces attention to the psychological aspects. It also withdraws attention from the processes which do not readily lend themselves to physiological treatment or do not fit into a physiological framework.

Thus a physiological psychologist like Thorndike has surprisingly little to tell us—even in his *Educational Psychology*, which would naturally consider matters obviously so important to an educationist—about volition or the creative imagination or the various aspects of emotions or sentiments, or even the development of character. And when we come to the subject of intelligence, our present topic, the distinctive quality of intelligence qua intelligence becomes invisible when viewed through physiological spectacles. Intelligence, with its intelligence left out, is readily reduced to a physiological formula. Reasoning appears as a case of stimulus and response—for association is only stimulus-response on the ideational level, one idea stimulating the arousal of another—' ideas ' are conveniently hypostatized for the purpose, and the one element in reasoning which accounts for degrees of native ability, namely the immediate *apprehension* of promising ' trial ' relations (hypotheses) and again of their relations to a series of actual situations (verification), goes unrecognized, since it does not fit into the physiological framework contrived to explain behaviour. Physiology is made master of psychology instead of its ally.

A further result of this physiological bias is the substitution of highly speculative and enigmatic physiological formulae for a plain statement of what actually occurs. Rather than admit the plain fact that superior native intelligence is signalized by a superior capacity in the individual for apprehending relations pertinent to purpose, and similarly of the relations of these relations to one another (integration), Thorndike prefers to transfer this power to the individual neurones, yet in such mysterious language as leaves us in some doubt as to just what he is attributing to them, or what part is played by the neurones and what by the individual's volition. In what respect is the simple psychological fact above referred to in any way *elucidated* by preferring the formula of " having the neurones act *in reference*

one to another, that is, with *integration* ? "[28]   Why not
give us the psychological fact, instead of a supposititious
and ambiguous physiological correlate ?   We all know
the educational precept "interpret the unknown by
means of the known"; here we have an educational
psychologist practising the opposite.

Now no one is more insistent than the trained
physiologist himself on our ignorance of the actual
physiological and neurological processes that correspond
with our conscious behaviour. " We do not know
exactly," writes C. J. Herrick, " how a sense organ is
excited, how a nerve fibre conducts, how a muscle
contracts, how a gland secretes, or how a brain thinks,
though we have satisfactory evidence that all of these
organs do perform the functions mentioned."[29]   Yet
we find an apologist for Thorndike's description of
intelligence with the temerity to claim that its special
superiority consists in its fitting so nicely the physiological facts.[30]

To summarize then the matter of this section : we
find Thorndike failing to do justice to the significance
of intelligence in human behaviour through his physiological predilections ; which lead him to ascribe some
peculiar efficacy to descriptions of psychological
phenomena in physiological language ; to mistake a
physiological correspondent of a psychological event
for the cause of that event ; to prefer a speculative
physiological to a plain psychological statement of a
psychological fact ; and to survey the psychological
region inadequately and out of perspective.   It ought
to be possible to absorb oneself in the physiology
of psychology without absorbing psychology into
physiology, though no doubt it demands some measure
of watchful detachment to do so.

IV. *Thorndike's Criticism of Intelligence as Relational
Thinking*

Of the view of intelligence as relational thinking

Thorndike disposes in a single page.[31] This dispatch of it seems to be due

(1) To a complete misunderstanding of the doctrine he is dismissing.

(2) To a confusion of associational and relational thinking. His confusion of the two is implied in the opening sentence of his criticism. " There is no doubt that the appreciation and management of relations is a very important feature of intellect, by any reasonable definition thereof."[32] One who maintains that the higher forms of intellectual operation are identical with mere association or connection forming and that the lower are also purely associative abilities can assign importance to relational thinking in intellect only by mixing up the two. In no other way can he admit relational thinking as " a very important feature " of the intellect and remain faithful to his associationist theory.

But it is also clear that he has failed to acquaint himself with the principles of the doctrine he sets out to attack. For he takes the doctrine to imply that " opposites and mixed relations tests " exemplify the perception and use of relations and " tests in paragraph reading, in information, and in range of vocabulary " do not. He also excludes from relational thinking " analysis (thinking things into their elements), selection (choosing the suitable elements or aspects of relations), and organizing (managing many associative trends so that each is given due weight in view of the purpose of one's thought) " which " seem as deserving of consideration as the perception and use of relations."[33]

But you do not discredit an opponent by demolishing a position he has never maintained. That the apprehension of relations is confined to opposites and mixed relations tests or to some faculty invoked on special occasions is an assumption of Thorndike's that the advocate of a relational concept of intelligence would not endorse for a moment. The theory that he purports to be rebutting maintains that *all mental cognitive process* involves the apprehension of relations and that individuals differ one from another in their ' apprehending ' ability, these differences yielding a criterion of what we may usefully call native intelligence. Barring mere sensation (if mere sensation ever occurs) some apprehension of relations is entailed in every concrete act of thinking, so that the mental operations at work in comprehending matter read, in getting information (it must be got in order to reproduce it), in reproducing vocabulary, and in analysis, selective thinking and organization, are not to be excluded. His criticism therefore is beside the point.

The doctrine held by Thorndike and the doctrine he professes to be attacking have this in common : both admit the existence of some unitary factor detectable at work in all cognitive processes. It is as to the nature of this factor that they disagree ; one claiming association, the other relational capacity, as the distinctive mark of intelligence in all mental process. Considering it is this very principle of the unitary factor that he has been notably contesting for many years in the doctrine he is now discussing (and which he has now himself espoused) his suddenly accusing it of not claiming to be unitary is inexplicable.

His next objection to the " relational thinking " theory is that it provides no criterion for grading intelligence. " Moreover," he writes, " I fear that in all our cases (namely relational thinking, analysis, selection, and organization) we need other valuations to decide which are the *better* relations or *more abstract* relations, or the *more essential* elements, or the *more sagacious* selection, or the *more consistent* organization, or the *more desirable* balance of weights, and the like."[34] Now even assuming this to be true of relational thinking, the question arises wherein does associational thinking admit valuation : which are the better associations or the more abstract associations, or the more desirable

associations, and so on.   In what way is the association
theory superior in this respect ?   In no way ; for the
association hypothesis of Thorndike expressly disavows
quality as a criterion of intelligence.   What right has
he therefore to disclaim the need of qualitative valuations
in his own doctrine but to require them in another ?

There is thus on his own premises no need to admit
his criticism as legitimate.   But assuming it legitimate,
a brief examination will show that it is invalid.   For
relational capacity does admit of degrees, degrees of
quality, enabling us to call A more intelligent than B.
It is indeed precisely the contrast between mere
associative thinking and relational thinking that yields
one criterion of superiority or inferiority of intelligence.
For there is no such thing as mere relational thinking
irrespective of an end or aim in view.   But the difference
between the inferior and the superior intelligence is in
proportion to the degree to which the individual thinker
approximates mere associative thinking on the one
hand (the " less intelligent " extreme) or thinks
relatively to purpose on the other (the " more intelligent "
extreme).   Now this is just the criterion that the
associative theory is by its very limitiatons precluded
from employing : it admits of no qualitative distinctions
whatsoever.   Thorndike has charged the alternative
doctrine with a defect which is conspicuously absent
from it, and conspicuously present in his own.   It is
the cardinal defect of his own doctrine.

The irrelevance of his criticism can only be ascribed
to failure to understand the position criticized.   This
failure is shown by his reading into the doctrine features
characteristic not of it but of his own ; so difficult is it
to detach oneself from one's established prepossessions.
Thus again we find Thorndike taking for granted that
the advocate of a ' relational 'theory must be judging
relational capacity by the number or quantity of
relations produced, or by the minimal stimulus required
to produce one.[35]   This is of course a travesty of the

theory : ' number ' may apply to the association theory, but the relational theory protests against this very view. *Relevance* is the important criterion. And the mere occurrence of a relation or a minimal stimulus is no guarantee of its quality.

In summary it may be claimed that Thorndike's criticism of the relational hypothesis of intelligence is based on misrepresentations or misunderstandings :

(1) It misunderstands the meaning of relational thinking altogether ;

(2) It wrongly assumes that relational thinking is a particular and not a general and unitary factor ;

(3) It mistakes it for a particular kind of *association* ;

(4) It wrongly assumes that it provides no criterion for distinguishing superior from inferior intelligence, a criterion which is lacking in his own doctrine. In fine it is not a criticism of the doctrine it purports to criticise ; and provides no reason for rejecting an alternative hypothesis of the nature of intelligence.

CHAPTER VII

INTELLIGENCE AND SPEARMAN'S CONCEPT OF 'G'

THE view of the nature of intelligence adopted in this treatise is in accord with the statistical and theoretical conclusions of two psychologists so different in their general doctrines as Thorndike and Spearman, in that intelligence is regarded as a native general ability which participates in all mental or at any rate all conscious cognitive process.

But it parts company with Thorndike and approaches much more nearly the position of Spearman in its account of what that common factor is   The operations of 'intelligence' it maintains cannot be explained as mechanical responses to stimuli, whether the stimuli be sensory stimuli, or (relaxing the rigour of the doctrine) 'ideas' or fragments of 'ideas' occasioned by sensory stimuli in the first instance.   Our doctrine, as against this, presumes the necessity of admitting an independent central power or faculty (there is no need to shun the word faculty), dependent for its material on what is supplied from 'experience,' but in the degree and efficiency of its exercise independent of the stimulus. There is, we suggest, intelligence, and there is as between individuals superior and inferior intelligence, other than mechanical reactions to stimuli or a capacity for a larger or lesser number of such reactions.

Further, this "central capacity," we suggest, is concerned particularly with the apprehension of relations between objects or 'ideas.'   For a mechanical bond is substituted a thought relation.

But the view of intelligence here offered differs from

the concept of ' g ' described by Spearman[1] in two main respects :

(1) The term intelligence in its purely cognitive aspect is reserved for the power of apprehending relations, as contrasted with the triple process indicated by ' g.'

(2) It is claimed that this power implied in intelligence is not just an apprehension of relations, it includes also relevancy of the relation to some object or end of which the individual is more or less aware. It is not the power of apprehending relations but the power of apprehending *pertinent* relations that constitute native intelligence in the most useful sense of the word, that in which individuals may be said to differ in intelligence.

It should be repeated before going further that of the two meanings attached to the term intelligence in popular discourse we are preferring to consider not a group of properties or innate attributes (sensory acuity, vitality, special tastes or aptitudes, physical strength or structure, disposition, temperament, and above all retentiveness) contributing to actual mental efficiency ; but a mental faculty, if there be one, distinguishable from these, which conditions mental efficiency in a high degree, is native, and not *in itself* susceptible of improvement, and distinguishes individuals as of higher or lower intelligence in a way that impresses the intelligent observer. We suggest that such a power exists and that the capacity to apprehend relations is that power.

One objection to the acceptance of ' g ' as equivalent to intelligence is that it involves an inconsistency.[2] Now ' g,' the common factor in cognition, is held by Spearman to correspond to three laws or processes. If these are independent of one another, if that is to say the power of individual A to exercise one of them better or worse than individual B is independent of his power to exercise the other two, then intelligence ceases to be a unitary factor. Instead of a single variable we have three independent variables, all claiming a share in intelligence, which is somehow constituted of all of them. Spearman will thus have abandoned his ' unitary' hypothesis. Further, he will have indicated three different criteria of intelligent activity, without attempting any comparative valuation of them. For in any concrete instance which of them is to have preference, and why ? Is A to be judged more intelligent than B if he knows his lived experience better, or if he educes relations better, or if he is better at educing correlates ?

But if on the other hand the three processes do not represent three different capacities, but superiority or inferiority in one process carries with it superiority or inferiority in the other two, the hypothesis of a unitary factor is preserved but we are left with the question, what is the unitary capacity common to all three, determining one's grade in all of them ? What is the single common factor ?

To this question Spearman gives no clear psychological answer.[3] Yet some kind of an answer is clearly demanded. Until we have one, his interpretation of his statistical results is incomplete : the statistics point to a single factor, the analysis to three.

So far as the problem of intelligence is concerned the answer to be here suggested is that the common factor is this relating capacity itself.

Spearman however denies this. For he has been careful to distinguish between these three laws of mental action or process, and protests against the suggestion that ' g ' measures the power to grasp relations.

" In the first place," he says, " such a formula would suggest only the educing of relations, and would therefore leave out of account the power—at least equally important—of educing correlates. In the second place, it would overlook the possibility, indeed probability, that ' g ' also enters into the power indicated by the first noegenetic law, that of knowing one's experience. Yet again, it would unjustifiably imply that ' g ' constitutes the *whole* of any such power, whereas the evidence indicates that ' g ' is never more than a factor in it."[4]

But if his arguments hold, the obvious retort to them is that we have in this case not arrived at ' g ' at all : the common factor which the statistics indicate and for which we have been so diligently searching is still missing. It is somewhere or other hidden amongst three processes, or it is more or less in all of them.

To the mind of the writer the problem does not seem so difficult of solution, nor the reasons for complicating it by this three-fold distinction convincing. Spearman appears to have been engaged in a logical rather than a psychological analysis. Logically the three processes are distinguishable, and for purposes of exposition it may be convenient to treat them separately. But surely the psychological function at work in all three is essentially the same, and it is in virtue of this identity of function that the first process occurs at all and that the third process performs its miracles.

Consider the first process : " Any lived experience tends to evoke immediately a knowing of its characters and experiences."[5] But surely in the nature of the case when we cognize or become aware of some lived experience—either sense data or affective or conative or volitional experience—our very becoming aware of it constitutes a relating. In the act of knowing it we no longer are it, we have detached ourselves from it and related it to ourselves as knowing. One may perhaps suffer a toothache without cognizing it ; whether that is possible or not is a moot question. But directly cognition comes in (the first glimmer of intelligence) the relating of the toothache to something not a toothache has appeared with it. To cognize an experience is to relate it. Our very first act of knowing is contrast. The point is made by the Gestalt psychologists when they note that the earliest conscious (in the sense of cognized) experience is of figure and ground. One cannot cognize a uniform continuum. Changelessness is incompatible with consciousness.

For this reason it is difficult to understand what different psychological process distinguishes the eduction of relations from the awareness of experience. The difference appears to be not in form but in matter.

The second formula, that of eduction of relations, runs as follows :

" The mentally presenting of any two or more characters (simple or complex) tends to evoke immediately a knowing of the relation between them."[6]

But all that has happened here is that the first process has been carried further. According to the first process characters have been discriminated, that is to say have been distinguished and related. For to distinguish is to relate.

Consciously to hold apart is to know as apart. We can then go on to establish further relations. The psychological process is the same : the relating.

But now let us take the third formula, the significance of which for the attainment of new knowledge, Spearman is at pains to emphasize, as also its irreducibility to the second process.

" The presenting of any character together with any relation tends to evoke immediately a knowing of the correlative character."[7]

Spearman maintains that whereas the second process is noegenetic in the sense that we become aware of a new relation (or of a relation of which we were previously unaware) the third process admits of our having an experience not previously experienced.

But whether Spearman does or does not succeed in making out his claim that by reason of this process we do arrive at new experience the point to be stressed here is that the appearance in consciousness of the correlate depends upon and is conditioned by the power of apprehending relations, and that whether the correlate will appear or not is directly dependent upon just that relating capacity. In other words it is the relating capacity that is the mental capacity involved ; the appearance of the correlative experience is its automatic outcome. Moreover what correlate will emerge depends upon what relation is held in consciousness, and it is just this ability to have and to hold a particular relation that constitutes the intelligence of the act. Holding one relation—the wrong one—, one,—the wrong—correlate will emerge ; holding the right one, the right correlate will emerge. The difference in intelligence between individuals is a difference in their capacity for apprehending the ' right ' relations. On this depends the ' intelligence ' of their response. For what is the process in detail ? It consists, as Spearman points out, in our being aware of a fundament and a relation ; on which the correlate tends to appear. The decisive factor here is clearly awareness of the relation. The fundament involves no special intelligence. And the appearance of the correlate is contingent on the relation having been apprehended. If this be granted, it would appear that it is in the power to grasp relations that intelligence as such resides.

To the three arguments advanced by Spearman in the passage just quoted the replies seem thus to be as follows : (1) That the formula " the power to grasp relations " does not in fact leave out of account the power to educe correlates, in as much as the power to educe correlates is itself consequent upon the power to educe relations, is indeed a practical outcome of it. (2) That the formula does not exclude the power to know one's own experience, in as much as knowing one's own experience is a case of apprehending relations and cannot take place without it.

There remains Spearman's third objection that the identifying of general intelligence with the power of relating would unjustifiably imply that ' g ' constitutes the *whole* of any such power whereas the evidence indicates that ' g ' is never more than a factor in it. The answer seems to be that in any specific case of relation educing it is impossible to make sure that other factors besides the mere relating do not come in, or to prove that the available statistical machinery is adequate to eliminate them ; so that we should hardly expect to find statistical ' g ' and the power to relate to be perfectly correlated. Spearman himself has given a number of reasons for not taking the statistical findings at their face value. It is however a noticeable support to our theory that, as Spearman points out, there is nothing to indicate that the different kinds of relations are unequal in respect of the degree that they make calls upon ' g.'

This brings us to the second main point of difference between intelligence and ' g.' The mere power to apprehend relations appears to be an inadequate description of general intelligence, in that it is necessary to add to the description the attribute of relevancy. The point is indeed implied by Spearman in his introductory chapter stating the problem when he says : " In general, a person's total cognitive ability may be regarded as an instrument or organ at the disposal of any of our conative activities."[8] But for purpose of logical treatment Spearman has deliberately left the conative aspect as far as possible out. Unfortunately this procedure, however convenient for preliminary exposition, misleads the students as to the bearing of conation upon the functioning, and the mode of functioning, of intelligence itself. By withholding from consideration the end or purpose of the individual, his desire or felt impulse or his intended objective, and by considering the intelligent activity in the abstract, the impression is produced that it is the objects of the cognitive consciousness, the fundaments of the noegenetic processes, that somehow generate and determine what relations shall arise. The reader finds himself framing a false picture of what actually in any concrete instance is taking place. According to the description, given fundaments are presented, and thereupon relations occur to us. It is as though the fundaments were capable of a number of fixed relations, had so to speak a certain repertoire of possible relations affixed to them or obtaining between them, and some or other of these proceed to emerge in consciousness. The terms of Spearman's formula supports this delusion. " The mentally presenting of any two or more characters tends to evoke immediately a knowing of relation between them."

But such a picture is misleading, for the intelligent relating activity is not just the relating as such. In the first place out of any number of characters presented relating will take place only between some of them. Some will escape unrelated. Birds are singing outside my study window, and within my study many sights assail my sense organs and pass the threshold of consciousness, yet no relations emerge between them. Meantime all sorts of relations are establishing themselves between characters of purely central origin. Furthermore the relations that do emerge are relations of a very particular kind or tendency. They are not just any relations set up by the fundaments alone. What governs the incidence of the relations, and the kind of relations that will occur between any objects of consciousness, is clearly not the mere existence of the fundaments, but the relevance of the fundaments themselves to some interest or end or purpose or objective which is at the time ' affecting ' me. Further again, the very appearance in consciousness of characters is not haphazard, but is itself conditioned by this very conative tendency. The intelligent operation does not go on, nor does it take the direction it does, merely in virtue of the pre-existence of the fundaments.

The bearing of this upon the activity of intelligence is exceedingly important. For the whole system of relations which is mentally set up is an intelligent system just in proportion to its general and particular relevancy to the end or purpose or ' motive.'

The whole picture or scheme or pattern of relations

or inter-relations is what it is and inter-related in the way it is because of the influence upon it of the end entertained. There is, so to speak, a general director, and the degree of intelligence which an individual exhibits in the case in question is proportioned to the degree (in fact *is* the degree) of his power to apprehend a whole act of interlaced relations all forming part of a single scheme. And the intelligent person is one who can display this gift of relevancy above the average. For this reason the term integration, or integration of relations, is really more illuminative than the term relating as such. The unintelligent person on the other hand is the person who lacks this power ; whose apprehended relations do not thus " hang together," or integrate into a pattern, but are relatively irrelevant, belong to several patterns, more or less discrepant with one another. The trouble about Spearman's purely intellectual consideration of intelligence is that it inevitably omits an indispensable feature of the picture, the most significant feature of it—the power of *relevancy*, of relating and inter-relating, of integrating, between the fundaments as a whole and some end " in view."

The difference between the unintelligent and intelligent individual is just that between two individuals, with equal intentness on the same end, and equal experience, of whom one can assemble the parts of an automobile so as to fit them into a whole machine and the other keeps bungling and fitting the wrong parts together. One apprehends the relevant relations, the other does not. He apprehends all sorts of relations which are relations no doubt but are not relevant.

We are ever acting analogously on the ideational plane. We are then said to think intelligently or unintelligently, or more generally to be intelligent or unintelligent people.

Summarily then native intelligence as here understood differs from Spearman's hypothesis of the psychological nature of ' g ' by way of subtraction and of supplement.

It subtracts from or is less than ' g ' in that it selects the power of apprehending relations as the essential factor common to the noegenetic processes, and identifies intelligence with that ; but it supplements ' g ' in adding to the concept the attribute of relevance, to some end or objective of which the individual is " more or less " aware.

It may help to clarify and confirm our hypotheses if reference is made to a few illustrations.

(1) From the field of animal psychology we may refer again to Köhler's apes. An ape that after a series of hesitant and unsuccessful movements in the general direction of his ' objective ' hits upon the practical solution by seizing a short stick and reaching with it for a long stick with which he then draws in the banana has done more than establish relations between a number of fundaments ; he has established such a series as " hangs together " and hangs together in a very particular way, namely in that way and that way only which is determined by the relation of the series to the final or end relation—the spatial conjunction of the ape and the banana.

(2) The ape who brings a box and holds it beneath the bananas suspended from the roof but is unable to mount the box because he is holding it has also apprehended relations and to some extent relevantly.[9] But he has failed to integrate the whole relational series. He has put together part of the situation but not the whole. To apprehend the whole series of relations in their relation to one another and to the end relation striven for would indicate a higher intelligence according to our hypothesis. But the creature displayed intelligence so far as it went.

(3) My little boy of two and half years of age has just been playing a simple card game with his mother. She puts on the floor in a row a card from each suit and while he watches attaches each card, as she draws it from

the pack, to the column of the corresponding suit. She then without a word of instruction lets him place each card as she hands it out. He does this correctly. In order to succeed he has had to apprehend relations of similarity and the general relation of these several relations to an end of view, namely attaching similars to similars.

(4) In one of Terman's intelligence tests for nine-year-olds the problem is to bring the words boy, ball, and river into a single sentence.

The child of ordinary intelligence has no difficulty : " The boy dropped his ball into the river," etc. But the mentally deficient child gives sentences like the following :

    a. A ball is for kicking.

    b. The boy goes and plays with another boy.

    c. Boys run.

And so on.[10]

In the one case the child has established a system of inter-related relations, and each relation established is relevant, or in relation to, the whole, and the whole, to the end in view, the creation of a sentence (itself a system of relations of a particular kind). But the deficient child has not " the intelligence " to integrate, that is to apprehend in one and the same act the relations within relations, to inter-relate and to apprehend just those relations which do relate not in a simple but in a multiple way. He apprehends a number of relations certainly, but he fails to apprehend those which relate to one another. The point which is illustrated is that any particular relation which arises is relevant not just to its particular immediate fundaments but at the same time to the system as a whole, that system again being related to the ' felt ' end.

(5) Take again an instance given by Spearman from analogies tests. " Prisoner is to jail as water is to : prison, drink, tap, bucket." " The correct completion,"

writes Spearman, " depends upon perceiving that the characteristic relation of a bucket to water is that of preventing its escape. This causal relation issues rationally from the essential natures of the related fundaments as ordinarily conceived. Accordingly—the answer ' bucket ' was given by almost all those testees who on independent grounds (confidential reports) had previously been rated as highly ' intelligent '; whereas the great majority of those who had been rated as ' unintelligent ' gave the answer ' drink '."*11

But in his analysis Spearman seems to miss the essential point. He represents the apprehension of the particular relation between prisoner and jail as *issuing from the nature of the related fundaments*, between which he asserts *the characteristic relation is that of preventing escape.*

But let us contrast the following :

' Prisoner ' is to ' jail ' as ' visitor ' is to : ' city,' ' prison,' ' hotel,' ' sight-seeing ? '   Surely the intelligent reader will have no difficulty in completing the analogy correctly.   But what has happened to the previously assumed " characteristic relation " ?   Another has taken its place.   And why ?   Because the particular relations apprehended between prisoner and jail, and again between the second set of fundaments, are conditional on the whole system of related fundaments and not on the items in detail.   The causal relation does not issue from the essential natures of the related fundaments, but from the end of the whole intellectual performance, which was in this case to discover two sets of relations which bear to one another the relation of similarity. By his failure to take the wider view Spearman has approached an absurdity.   For who can reasonably

*This instance supports the suggestion that it is the relation held in consciousness which determines the correlate, and the ' intelligence ' of that correlate.   The superior testee answers ' bucket ' because he has the right relation in mind, the inferior ' drink ' because he is carrying another.   The superiority of intelligence in Speakman's third process therefore resides within the relating, not in the effecting of the correlate.

claim that preventing escape is the characteristic relation of ' bucket ' to ' water.' Far more characteristic is the relation of " containing it." We do not ordinarily in using pots and pans regard them as preventing the escape of what is in them but of containing or holding them ; and the only reason why this particular relation occurs to the intelligent testee on this occasion is not because it is the relation which issues rationally from the essential natures of the fundaments as ordinarily conceived but because it is the relation which fits the whole system of fundaments in their relation to the felt end. In other words it is not in apprehending separate relations on their own merits that intelligence resides but in the capacity to apprehend or select that relation which fits a purposed system or a dominant design. The determinant is primarily subjective—the end in view—not the nature of the fundaments as ordinarily conceived. Rather it is the nature of the fundaments as *specially conceived for the object at the moment.*

The characteristic quality of intelligence, as these illustrations indicate, is not the power to relate as such nor the tendency of lived experience to evoke relations between isolated fundaments, nor yet the tendency for a relation and a fundament or relations and fundaments to evoke correlates, but the capacity of the individual to apprehend as between any number of presented fundaments a system of relations, the capacity to integrate objects of consciousness coherently, to become aware of those relations and just those relations which do so cohere, the coherence being again not mere coherence, but coherence or consonance with some more or less clearly ' intended ' end.

We may usefully conclude this chapter by reverting to some of the most typical current definitions of intelligence which call attention to one or other of its practical outcomes or attributes, and tracing their relations to the central common psychological factor.

Consider the five following renderings of intelligence,

which seem on the face of them noticeably different from one another :

(1) The power of good responses from the point of view of truth or practice.

(2) The power of adjusting or adapting to novel circumstances.

(3) The acquiring faculty.

(4) The power to profit by experience.

(5) The power of abstract or of conceptual thinking.[12]

A brief analysis will show that, except the last, which alone is a psychological definition, they are various statements of certain practical consequences or effects of the exercise of a single common psychological power or process, namely that of apprehending relevant relations ; and that *this* is the common element which harmonizes their apparent variety. To take them *seriatim.*

Presumably by the power of good responses from the point of view of truth or practice is meant the power to answer truly or to act efficiently, for what else can be intended ? Now we may answer truly, that is correctly, either because we have been correctly informed and remember accurately, or because we "immediately apprehend" the correct answer. The first involves intelligence but in a comparatively low degree, since it depends upon retentiveness very largely and upon information. But even here some intelligence comes in : for in order to answer a question on matter learnt it is necessary not only to recall something retained, but to recall an experience related to the intention of the question, and in that relation. Moreover some intelligence, that is some apprehension of relations, entered into the original understanding of the information given. To be able to answer correctly in the second case contemplated of course involves intelligence in a higher degree, for it depends upon one's effecting a certain relation for the first time there and then.

Again, to act efficiently or to respond well from the point of view of practice (that is as the occasion requires, or as one's needs suggest), entails precisely the power to relate. Köhler's apes furnish abundant examples. Or consider a child building his castle of bricks. If he rightly apprehends the relation of position and size and shape beforehand, or as he goes along, he will build the more efficiently; if he trust merely to trial and error, the less. So with an architect planning a house or an administrator solving a practical human problem. Of course in every concrete case in actual life factors besides intelligence make a great deal of difference. No one would deny this. All that is maintained is that of two architects planning the same kind of house in otherwise identical conditions, the one who plans the more efficiently is he who in planning or executing the building can apprehend the relations obtaining between the different parts and processes of the building and can frame " in his head " a scheme with its parts inter-related so as to form a harmonious whole. In other words he must be able to apprehend a set or system of relevant relations, all ' integrated ' in their relation to his main purpose, or final or end relational system. That and just that is the contribution of intelligence to efficient action, to the excellence of one's response in a practical situation.

From this it will follow also that the power to adapt or adjust to novel circumstances is *ceteris paribus* just this power of relevant apprehension. The individual who in a strange situation, say in a new country, is likely to get on best is, *ceteris paribus*, he who in a social situation, instead of acting just habitually, apprehends the etiquette and manners of his new acquaintances, that is, can relate a particular action to the elements of the situation to which it does relate, and can then go on to apply, that is to apprehend, a similar relation on another occasion. Moreover he systematizes (that is apprehends in their relations to one another) a large number of specific particular relations, and so gradually effects his adjustment.

The "acquiring power" clearly depends upon the same faculty. Apart from retentiveness and mere reproduction the acquiring of any new skill or knowledge entails an apprehension of new relations, and their embodiment in practice. Even so simple a skill as working the gears of an automobile depends primarily upon the power to relate one movement to another—one must first apprehend the temporal relation of the different movements before embodying it in practice. Whereon practice (or repetition dependent on retention) confirms the skill. Now such simple motor skills do not correlate highly with general intelligence. And this is just what we should expect. For though they depend upon the apprehension of relations, the establishment of the skill depends also very largely upon purely physiological attributes—those facts of bodily structure which underlie efficient muscular co-ordination and are not in themselves expressions of intelligence. Consequently some but not high correlation with the criterion might be anticipated.

Again in successful profiting from experience it is experience (previous performance or knowledge) that furnishes the fundaments ; profiting by the use of them is dependent upon effecting relations between them. To profit by experience is not of course the mere rein-stating of some previous knowledge or performance : that depends upon retention with reproduction, and by itself would result in stereotyping performance and not in progress. But repeated repetition, since it decreases demand for effort, releases energy for establishing new relations between the represented fundaments, and it is here that progress comes in. To profit from experience means then :

(1) Reinstatement of past knowledge or performance, with added facility of performance and less energy expenditure ; and a

(2) Consequent greater chance of apprehending new relations between the objects presented. Thus new fundaments in the shape of the new relations replace or embrace the old.

The added facility it may be noted is signalized by an increasing clarification or distinctness of the fundaments, analogous to the growing distinctness of the different parts of a scene as we continue to gaze at it. It is perhaps this " separating out " of the elements which renders them easier to relate.

We now come to the description of intelligence as the power of abstract or conceptual thinking. Here we have a psychological definition of a psychological capacity ; and in so far as relational thinking becomes increasingly difficult, and therefore a severe test of intelligence or a test of superior intelligence, the more remote from the original sense-given fundaments the operations go on, to that extent the definition provides an approximately accurate criterion. But a criterion is not thereby identical with its object.

In the first place, the term abstraction is too ambiguous and comprehensive. All relating no doubt involves abstracting, for we relate fundaments to one another only in virtue of certain common properties which must therefore first be ' abstracted,' in the sense of being " separately intended " or attended to. But the converse need not be true ; an abstraction need not be a relating. An image, for instance, is an abstraction—it is not the concrete thing it stands for, but a mentally abstracted semblance or partial semblance of it.

Secondly, the definition lays stress upon one incident of the " intelligent act " rather than upon the act itself. In the act of intelligence the abstracting is subordinate to, and determined by, the relevant relating, and not *vice versa*. As has already been pointed out, the relating process is itself relevant to some end or final relation striven for, and any abstraction that takes place is nothing more nor less than the mental intending or discriminating of such aspects or attributes of presented fundaments as serve the relation determined by the final objective.

Thirdly, the power to think abstractly may suggest, and to most readers probably does suggest, the power to think in the absence of the concrete. The power to apprehend relations conveys no such suggestion. Now degrees of intelligence, or of facility in apprehending relations are exhibited just as much when applied to perceptual fundaments, as when we are " thinking abstractly " or on the ideational plane. I may not only handle perceptual situations, I may even perceive objects, more or less intelligently, according as I apprehend the relations they admit of more or less readily and relevantly. Contrast an ape, a child, and a mature human intelligence dealing with Sultan's perceptual problems. For the same reason intelligence cannot be identified with the power of thinking conceptually, since thinking perceptually involves intelligence also.

PART II

CHAPTER VIII

INTELLIGENCE AND INSTINCT

THERE have been many discussions of the relation between intelligence and instinct, especially in the last twenty years, and the subject might be considered threadbare. But there are special reasons for reconsidering it here. For though such discussions have been preceded by, and have assumed, a concept of instinct based upon a more or less adequate analysis, they have been largely handicapped by a certain vagueness as to the psychological connotations of the term intelligence. And they have in fact themselves as a rule been devoted much more to clarifying their author's conceptions of instinct than in elucidating intelligence, which is disposed of in general terms such as adaptation to new circumstances or reinstatement of experience, etc., without any adequate indication of how this adaptation takes place or what mental processes are involved in effecting it. It is however not possible to map out the respective areas of instinct and intelligence in human behaviour until we have decided what psychological processes correspond to both the terms.

As a provisional hypothesis of intelligence has already been advanced, it is necessary briefly to indicate the particular meaning to be ascribed to the term instinct. This will be done somewhat dogmatically to avoid a treatment of instinct disproportionate to the object in view.

One of the reasons for the current controversy over the character and scope of instinctive factors in human behaviour is that overt instinctive behaviour is so differently manifested in the upper and lower grades of the evolutionary scale of life as to obscure its fundamental unity. Contrast for example the instinct of fear or escape as exhibited in man with the following instance of instinctive activity in a comparatively low grade of animal life.

" The Yucca moth emerges from the chrysalis when the Yucca flower is in bloom. The moth flies to the Yucca flower, collects pollen from its anthers and kneads it into a pellet, and flies with this to another bloom, the pistil of which she pierces with her ovipository lancet, and lays her eggs among the ovules. Then, darting to the top of the stigma, she stuffs the fertilizing pollen pellet into its funnel-shaped opening. This elaborate performance, which she has never herself witnessed, takes place once for all."[1]

How widely different is man's behaviour in securing and safe-guarding the arrival of his progeny, and how various in detail. So various that many psychologists in searching for the common minima reduce them to certain concatenations of reflexes, or hereditary behaviour patterns (irrespective of accompanying perception, impulse and emotion), and have consequently identified instinct with these mechanical universals ; or have gone to the extreme of rejecting human instincts altogether.

This is not the view taken here. Instinct undoubtedly differs widely in its manifestations in human and, let us say, insect life ; so widely as to warrant differences in the definition of the term as between the species at different ends of the evolutionary scale, though sufficiently alike in essential features to yield a definition of general applicability. In the case of the insect, for example, instinctive behaviour may be defined as an activity (adaptive and common in its essentials to the species) consisting of a performance whole or series, executed apart from experience, arising on each occasion in certain like circumstances, concluding in certain like ends, and comprising a succession of like intermediate units ; apparently prompted by impulse and accompanied by some degree of consciousness and sustained by endeavour.

Compare and contrast with this a definition of instinct in man : " An innate disposition which common to a species determines the organism apart from experience to perceive or attend to certain inner conditions or external objects of a certain class, to experience accordingly a certain emotional excitement and an impulse to carry through some action (which is on the whole adaptive) in relation to that object or those conditions."[2]

The common factors in the two definitions are universality, adaptiveness, independence of experience, but dependence for arousal on certain experiences of the organism itself.

But there are important differences : in insect instinct there is emphasized the fixed and complex performance series, contrasting with the marked variety of human behaviour ; and in man the prominence of the conscious states of impulse and emotion, as contrasted with the appearance only of some degree of impulse and excitement in the insect.

Another point may be added—the insect often exhibits far more *apparent* persistence than the man. Remove for the ammophila wasp the prey from before its hole again and again, and again and again the wasp proceeds to replace it as before.[3]

As already mentioned, the fact that the overt behaviour presents so little uniformity in man has frequently led to a denial of its instinctive character. But in so rejecting or belittling instinct in man the point of the contrast between human and insect instinct has been missed. The difference in the two cases is not that the one grade of instinct lacks the uniformity which marks the other, but that the uniformity is differently located.

In the insect the uniformity is that of objective performance, and therefore easily observable ; but in man it is uniformity of impulse or emotion, which are subjective and in their nature not directly observable,

but none the less equally uniform and universal
Psychology has been apt to miss instinct in man because
it has been seeking only for uniformities of overt
behaviour : it has forgotten that they might be of
another kind, less open to direct observation.

Further, it is just because the problem has been
approached without a clear psychological conception
of intelligence that the difficulty of reconciling instincts
so differently manifested has arisen ; and the underlying
identity has been overlooked. For in the light of our
present hypothesis of intelligence the differences are
not only explicable, but precisely the differences one
would have expected to find. It would have been
strange if there had been no such contrasts.

The explanation here suggested for the differences
is that in the course of evolution of living organisms
instinct itself has developed, and in the direction of
intelligence. As we pass from chapter to chapter in
the story of life, we find instinct itself becoming ever
less blindly impulsive, and more emotional; less
mechanical, and more conscious ; less determined, and
more intelligent. The three contrasts are different
aspects of one general development ; they have
co-operated with one another. But our immediate
interest is to confine our attention to the growing
incidence of intelligence in the evolutionary process,
and to trace its bearing on the evolution (not on the
elimination) of instinct.

The development of intelligence within instinctive
behaviour has followed three distinguishable lines :

(1) In environmental range of application ;

(2) In freedom or expansion within the range of the
particular instinct itself ;

(3) In level of consciousness at which it functions.
To explain and illustrate *seriatim*.

An outstanding difference between man and the lower
animals is in range of instinctive interest. The worm,
the ant, the bird, the dog, are limited by endowment

to a very narrow range of activities, so that it is possible to comprise within a small compass the life story of any one of them. Their lives are in the main prescribed and delimited for them by heredity. The bee pays no attention to the bone, nor the dog to the fragrant flower. Their intelligent activity—the power of apprehending relations—is limited correspondingly. Intelligence is imprisoned within boundaries set by instinct. There is no impulse to exercise intelligence beyond them. At the grade of development nearest— in present species—to that of man there has been a marked expansion of the boundaries, witness the play activities, and the curiosity, of Köhler's apes ; but even in the apes these instinctive boundaries are fairly clearly marked. Intelligence remains the servant of instinctive impulse. The evolutionary gap between even the highest apes and man is wide. Yet it represents a continuity, not a break, in development. By original nature man also is a creature of instinct and exercises his intelligence within instinctive boundaries. Of this initial limitation he is largely unaware ; for four reasons :

a. A reason residing within the nature of instinct itself, since, by confining attention within its own limits, it precludes awareness of what is beyond them ; and, therefore, of its own limitations. For we do not recognize the significance of what we do not observe.

b. When the evolutionary human plane of development has been reached, the range of instinctive activities has so far widened beyond that of the lower animals that the comparative psychologist is struck more by the width and variety of a child's activities than by their limitations. Their variety strikes him because the lower animals are always with us ; but not their limitations, for we meet no angels.

c. The enlarged participation of intelligence in instinctive behaviour lends to it such variety as to obscure both its real character and the limits within which that variety is confined.

H

Lastly, and most important of all,

d. Once it attains (phylogenetically) a certain level of development, intelligence evolves the means of its own freedom. Man alone can intelligently acquire control of instinct.* This very fact, of course, is evidence of the existence of that which is controlled ; but the consequent difference in the status of instinct in animal and man is so marked as to lead many to under-rate the very large influence instinct still exerts upon human conduct.

Since, then, at the human stage in evolution the range of instinctive activities has greatly widened, the range of intelligent activities has widened with it. In man impulses to narrow lines of behaviour are comparatively few. He is concerned by nature with more general ends. His intelligence is more widely exercised accordingly.

This brings us to the second line of development of intelligence in instinctive behaviour. In the lower animal the instinctive performance is so narrowly prescribed, so fixed in detail, as to present relatively few opportunities for the exercise of intelligence. Each complex performance series is linked up by many unit performances or subordinate ends, consists of a series of landmarks, as it were, each not distant from its predecessor, and requiring but a low level of intelligence to bridge the interval. The bird's nest-building, and its mating performances comprise each a succession of unit performances within the wholes, performances hereditarily determined and less precise than the action series of the Yucca moth, but more precise than the instinctive performances of man. So uniform are these series that there is no need to suppose the bird has any foresight of the end (the completed nest) when she begins to fetch the straws ; for each completed unit

---

*But even animals do learn to control impulse intelligently (see p. 34) ; but the difference of degree in this respect between the highest animals and man is immense.

leads on to, inaugurates the next. And so with the courting and mating behaviour of birds. It is all describable in fairly uniform terms.

With this let us compare and contrast human courtship and mating. Here the main lines of the process are also instinctively determined. The mating impulse is a powerful hereditary instinct—so powerful that society has imposed conventional checks upon it. The mating act with which it concludes is essentially the same. And the intermediate stages—the approach and display of the male, the coyness and receptivity of the female, the types of behaviour providing cumulative stimulus— these have their prototypes in the more precise perform-ances of lower animals ; from which (or rather from collateral ancestors) they derive. But contrast the scope for intelligence. In the animal behaviour impulse predominates. He goes mostly unthinkingly ahead. Instinct seems almost enough. But in the human suitor instinctive impulse and intelligent direction are inextricably mixed. The sexual urge, and its accom-panying emotion, are strongly marked. Their influence is insistent, sometimes so insistent that intelligence is exercised only in planning satisfaction. And plan it does. The youth thinks ahead how he may again meet the maiden, considers ways of finding favour in her eyes, of arousing a return of his ardour, and of winning her submission or assent. So far as the purely instinctive factors are concerned intelligence co-operates with instinct at every step ; and discovers a wide variety of alternative and successive relations, and again of the relations between these and the end in view. The capacity to apprehend more than mere impulse supplies is the capacity of intelligence. The youth's behaviour is indirect and varies accordingly. But it is none the less instinctive. The impulse, the emotion, the end are not of his devising—they happen to him, they are part of his nature. Within the limits they prescribe intelligence has ample play. Thus in its freedom or

scope within the instinct itself the intelligence of man
has advanced immensely upon the beast.

Thirdly there is an advance in the level of consciousness at which intelligence functions.

Consider the intermediate level, represented, say, by
the chimpanzee. So far as Köhler's observations went,
the apes were able to apprehend relations mainly within
(or scarcely beyond) the immediate perceptual field
(namely of vision), though cases were cited in which
an ape did include within the reach of its thinking an
object remembered but not actually present. Sultan
apprehended the bearing of objects and places (not
within immediate range of vision) upon the position of
the objective to be secured.[4] Apes who had seen food
buried in a certain spot the day before, but had had no
access to it, were able 17 hours after, when the spot
came into the visual field again, to recall a previously
apprehended relation, and to act accordingly. They
were thus capable of some measure of ' tied ' ideation.

But between these achievements and the human power
of thinking freely, of reproducing situations, with no
part of them objectively present, and of apprehending
relations between elements within those situations, or
between one situation or part situation and another,
the evolutionary interval may be wider than that
between the highest of the apes and the lowest grade of
animalcule. Yet the principles of intelligence and of
instinct are the same. So too the solitary ammophila
wasp which normally stamps and rolls flat the dirt over
her hole with her feet, but on one occasion is seen to
use a pebble for the purpose, is capable of apprehending
a hitherto unrecognized relation ;[5] so too was the sphex
wasp that omitted one step in its instinctively prescribed
ritual, and instead of dropping the paralysed caterpillar
just outside its home while she went down it and came up
again, after the observer had repeatedly removed her
prey to a distance, at last altered her behaviour and
carried the caterpillar immediately into the nest. She

could so far apprehend the relation of her two acts to one another as to be able to unite them into one, and to supersede instinct.

But there is no need to select specially striking instances. The co-operation of intelligence with instinct is observable at every turn. The dog that runs round a tree to fetch a bone that lies on the other side—instead of hitting against the trunk ; or so manipulates a bone as to place it more conveniently for biting, is not acting mechanically ; he is or contains no machine for adapting to each novel situation of its own accord. For machines do not adapt to each novel situation of their own accord : they have only a fixed set of quite uniform reaction patterns. The dog is at least intelligent enough to apprehend, within a very near perceptual situation, certain relatively simple relations between objects, and to act accordingly.

Thus we claim that every living organism is intelligent in its degree : that intelligence is implicit in organic life as such. It is the principle in virtue of which the organism is not a machine : it is life's distinctive quality. There is no point in the scale at which it suddenly comes in.

Nor is it difficult to suggest certain differences in the limits of consciousness which accompany and condition the evolutionary progress of intelligence. The human intelligence is especially competent to do this, in that— on the highest development of intelligence—it comprehends or includes actually (and so can comprehend intellectually) every stage that went before it. It functions, that is to say at every degree and level up to the limit attained by itself. To represent or to experience—to ' empathise '—the particular level of consciousness which accompanies in a dog or an insect intelligent activities of the creature's appropriate level, the human intelligence must revive or recall its own level of consciousness when engaged in activities of the same intelligence level.

For instance man is capable of ' free ' ideation because he can ' freely ' remember.   He cannot sit and consider that which he cannot recall.   On the other hand man can, and does, act upon an idea which he has never even made explicit in consciousness.   The ' idea ' was sufficiently " in consciousness " to affect action, but not to ensure its own reproduction nor even its conveyance to others.   To be able to communicate an ' idea ' to another in verbal language consciousness must be ' explicit,' one's awareness must be definite and differentiated—each element in the general impression must be distinguished and held apart.   We know the difficulty of " having an idea," but being unable to express it. But we also know that we can, and do, act upon it when it is in that undifferentiated and implicit state.   And we know that state ; it is a common human experience.

The point of interest here is that that experience, that state of implicit consciousness, seems to be all that the animal usually, and in lower grades of animal life ever requires for the levels of intelligent activity to which it attains.   That then is all we need postulate for it.   It does not communicate in language ; it shows scant evidence of free ideation—that clear and distinct and vivid analytic consciousness which conditions in man verbal communication and free ideation need not be assumed in the lower animal.   But that low level of awareness of what we are doing as we avoid a stone in our path or step off the side-walk, or return to our hotel in a newly visited city, without noticing our direction, by the way by which we came, that we may assume, say, in the dog, because movements of that level of intelligence are its ordinary repertoire.   Such consciousness may be fleeting, implicit, and confined to perceptual situations as distinct from our sustained, explicit, and ideational awareness when we are engaged in thinking out a problem in solitude, or in planning some project, or in putting our ideas into suitable words.

A caution is necessary to make clear that the emotional

consciousness is not being considered here. The emotional consciousness of the animal may be intense ; that is a separate question. But its cognitional consciousness, on the principle of economy of consciousness, need not be assumed so. Summarily then while we find the principle of intelligence in all grades of living organism, it functions in the lower grades in a far narrower range of activities, within narrower limits within these activities, and on a lower and less explicit conscious level.

We are now in a position to attempt an answer to the question whether intelligence itself is not an instinct, for several authors think that it is. Our answer to this question will throw light on another question of paramount psychological importance—whether intelligence is the servant or director of instinctive impulse in man.

The claim that intelligence is instinctive has been supported by a formidable array of arguments,[6] which may be briefly enumerated :

(1) Intelligence is admittedly innate.

(2) It is in degree universal to the species, or at least as general as any ordinarily accepted instinct is. The exceptional feeble-minded person is paralleled by the exceptional individual in whom some instinct (e.g. the sex instinct or the instinct of fear) is of minimal intensity.

(3) It exists also, though no doubt in a lesser degree, in the lower animals. This is one of the criteria of instinct.

(4) It is capable of perversion (e.g. lying), as are the other instincts. Witness the evidence of abnormal psychology. Existence in markedly abnormal forms is another criterion of instinct.

(5) It functions for the first time apart from previous training, and apparently spontaneously. The infant thinks without being taught to do so. We all browse and day-dream more or less.

(6) It is adaptive—favouring self-preservation or race-preservation. So is instinct.

(7) It has its appropriate emotional accompaniment : the glow of satisfaction with successful exercise of intelligence. Instinct has also its appropriate emotional accompaniment.

(8) Baulked it gives rise to annoyance. It is a mark of instinct that when thwarted the emotion of anger arises.

(9) The process of intelligent activity is a unit performance with a certain series of recognizable steps— the occurrence of a hypothesis, its trial, its rejection or selection, and so on. Instincts also function in certain unit series.

(10) Its functioning is prompted by a certain specific class of situation or object, namely, the encountering of the ' novel ' or unfamiliar. To be aroused by certain particular conditions or objective stimuli is a mark of instinct.

In the face of such a set of more or less convincing arguments it would seem difficult to reject intelligence from the category of instincts.

Objections to some of these arguments will have occurred to the reader ; but the simplest and shortest way of dealing with them is perhaps not to attempt to evaluate or counter them in detail, but to confront them with an alternative position :

(1) Intelligence is in a different category from instinct altogether. It is an instrument or capacity and not in itself an impulse or force. We can no more claim it as an instinct than we can claim the power of vision, or the capacity for discriminating sounds, as instinctive, though both are innate, universal to the species, varying in degree between individuals, adaptive, found in the lower animals, and when exercised, accompanied by some kind of affective tone ; and when exercised unsuccessfully, proportionately annoying to the organism. The processes of seeing and hearing are also analyzable into uniform steps or units. Both function apart from experience.

But to designate every innate capacity as instinctive on these grounds is to deprive instinct of its distinctive significance.

(2) Intelligence admittedly is closely associated with instinctive activity—it is indeed a capacity utilized by every instinct which cannot attain its object by the direct movement of impulse. Impulse moves primarily directly to its end. Bar its way, and either failure *or* intelligence supervenes. The latter, however, not by any force of its own, but impelled by the instinct, whose instrument it is. In other words the organism experiences an alternative impulse—towards the object, or to the exercise of intelligence if the object is not directly attained.

On this view the cardinal differences between intelligence and instinct are that intelligence is a capacity, and not a pre-disposition to act upon an impulse, and that it reacts to no specific situation peculiar to itself, since it functions in the service of any instinct, and under the impulsion of that instinct. Nor is it, like instincts in general, an hereditary determiner of behaviour.

In thus stating the case we must however avoid the error of passing from one extreme position to the other. It will be necessary presently to advance certain qualifications of our general statement, by admitting a certain sense in which intelligence may be regarded as instinctive, provided we interpret the term instinctive a little liberally.

But first another argument for the instinctive character of intelligence may be met, namely, that which associates it particularly with the instinct of curiosity. The contention is that animals and man experience an impulse to investigate a novel object, provided however the object is not too novel, when it provokes the instinct of fear. Wonder is the appropriate emotion, and the understanding of the object the end.

" The native excitant of the instinct," says McDougall, " would seem to be any object similar to, but perceptibly different from, familiar objects habitually noticed. It is therefore not easy to distinguish in general terms between the excitants of curiosity and those of fear ;

for we have seen that one of the most general excitements of fear is whatever is strange or unfamiliar. The difference seems to be mainly one of degree, a smaller element of the strange or unusual exciting curiosity, while a larger or more pronounced degree of it excites fear."[7]

To admit such a separate instinct however is to duplicate unnecessarily the course of intellectual activity, which has already been claimed as derivable from the impulse embodied in every instinct to exercise intelligence when hindered from attaining its end immediately. Now the arousal of the impulse in instinct follows upon a certain mental activity, namely the perception of an object or situation. But what is perception? It is the process of apprehending an object or situation as of a certain class; and after the instinct has been once aroused such classification is in future cases the normal precedent of instinctive activity. Perception is the interpretation of an object. Interpreting the object in one way, for instance, the horse shies; in another way, it passes the object with indifference. In many, possibly in most instances, the perception preliminary to the arousal of the instinctive activity presents no difficulty; the perception is practically immediate, and the appropriate instinctive activity follows.

But exceptions are not uncommon—perception may be hesitant, uncertain. The object is not of a familiar class. The animal proceeds to inspect it diffidently, or, if a domesticated animal unused to danger, greets it with a prolonged stare. If then the object is perceived as of the class dangerous, there follow the instinctive expressions of fear. There is of course no objection to applying the term curiosity to this tentative probing, nor, perhaps, to designating the emotion as wonder. But surely it is more properly described as the preliminary phase in the functioning of any instinct where the percept is ambiguous, than as a separate instinct functioning in its own right.

Thus, briefly, there are two places in the course of instinctive behaviour where intelligent activity is provoked, one in the endeavour to satisfy a checked instinctive impulse, the other, in cases of doubtful perception, in the preliminary stage.

On this principle is explained—a point not explained by McDougall—why the novel object sometimes provokes curiosity, sometimes fear. It provokes fear directly it is perceived as of a dangerous nature ; it provokes curiosity before it is adequately perceived at all.

Moreover the " separate instinct " hypothesis fails to explain why and at what point the curiosity will be satisfied. If an animal has an instinct of investigation why should the instinct function only in the presence of the unfamiliar, and why should the ' curious ' creature not pursue his inquiries indefinitely ? The alternative hypothesis has a ready answer to both these questions The novel arouses curiosity because it is not yet perceived (or classified) and curiosity ceases as soon as it ceases to be novel ; as soon, that is, as it falls into a recognizable class. The end or objective is not disinterested discovery (which a separate instinct of curiosity implies), but the animal's immediate welfare, the recognition of the meaning of the object in ' instinct-arousing ' terms. Thus the instinct of curiosity resolves itself into a part activity of other instincts. Most instances of animal curiosity appear to be covered by these conditions ; just as in most cases animal intelligence functions in the service of instinct (whether in the preliminary or the intermediate stage).

But perhaps not all. And here we may withdraw a little from the extreme position provisionally adopted. The doctrine of specific instincts does not suffice to cover all human, nor indeed all animal, activities. Life has one characteristic apt to be overlooked if we narrow our view too severely to a set of particular impulses provoked by a series of particular objects or situations. For supposing the particular objects are not present.

The organism does not cease to exist. Far otherwise. It may have satisfied its hunger and its thirst and its sexual cravings, have nothing particular about it to provoke anger or fear or submission or self-assertion or acquisitiveness or indeed any instinct in particular. It is free from environmental pressure of any specific kind. And, let us assume, it is not fatigued enough to sleep or rest. Yet the animal not only continues to exist, it continues to be *active*. The one fundamental fact of life—the great non-specific general instinct (if we may now so stretch the word) is *activity* itself. Activity goes on even when *instincts* are not specifically stimulated.

This characteristic of life provides a clue to ' play.' Play is activity in the absence of instinctive urgencies. (In man of course, in the absence of acquired urgencies as well). The form which such activity will take—the particular activities—are conditioned by the organism's endowment, its capacities and its sense-organs. In its ' spare ' periods the organism if not fatigued—exercises its capacities by means of its sense organs in relation to its environment. One could hardly expect it to do anything else. But the matter does not rest here. For though there may be no instinctive urge, and no particularly provocative situation, yet every instinctive performance obeys the law of re-instatement of experi-ence—it tends to its own repetition, to beget a habit, or (to reserve the term habit to a narrower usage) a disposition to recurrence. The ' spare ' periods of the organism—free from serious stimulation—are thus largely occupied in ' mock ' instinctive activities, with no serious intent, and on the merest symptom of provocation ; in other words in play. It is therefore a mark of play that the instinctive performance is not carried through to its genuine, serious, or adaptive end. The reason is plain : there is no *serious* specific stimulus, no real provocation, no actual need. The instinct is merely functioning through force of habit ; or—even apart from habit—through force of the instinct itself, on a mere hint of a stimulus, when no strong urge or need is present. Thus the unchained house dog ' plays '—but the chained dog (its urge unsatisfied) is more likely to bark than to play. Play is a function of contentment. The discontented human only affects to play.

Incidentally it may be noted how the trite ' theories ' of play fall into line under this principle. The activity may be regarded as superfluous, if we mean by superfluous not occupied in the satisfaction of specific instinctive needs, but it is not superfluous in the sense of being extra to the organism's ordinary occupations. It may be regarded as preparatory, in the sense of exercising the organism in movements useful in the serious business of life, but it is not preparatory in the sense of being undertaken primarily *for that object*. Again, it is recapitulatory, in the sense of repeating the activities of its forebears, but it is not recapitulatory in the sense of being determined in kind and sequence primarily by the order of appearance in the race.

To evaluate the various theories of play is not, however, our present purpose ; which is to indicate the bearing of this discussion upon the part taken by intelligence in animal and particularly human life. For in the first place the exercise of intelligence will appear in con- junction with ' playful ' instinct in this ' leisure ' life ; for it is part of instinctive activity. But—and this is the important qualification—since in play the ' instinc- tive ' end is neither urgent nor insistent, its hold upon intelligence itself is proportionately relaxed, and intelligence itself is proportionately free. The habit or disposition of intelligent exercise formed in the stern service of some compelling urge reappears when the genuine urge is absent, but for that very reason, is not tied to a single or dominant end.

And so far as the level or limits of intelligent capacity admit, even an animal can exhibit some independent play (or display) of intelligence in less occupied moments.

Hence the more or less intelligent play of Köhler's apes ; and hence the many instances of so-called ' curiosity ' in the higher animals, in the absence of any imperative instinct. They were following what may better be called general tendencies, rather than any instinct of curiosity in particular.

The following propositions may serve as summary :

(1) Intelligence appears as the servant and assistant of instinct, both in the preliminary stage where perception is incomplete, and in the intermediate stage of endeavour to satisfy the impulse.

(2) There is no need to postulate a separate instinct of curiosity ; but

(3) In the form of play or in periods not dominated by instinctive stress the organism may display the freer intelligent concern in its surroundings, whether as playful independent exercise or as part of a play instinctive process.

So far then we have been treating in this chapter the functioning of intelligence in the instinctive stage of animal and human life. But, as the human individual develops, he becomes capable of professional or of a disinterested pursuit of truth ; and intellectual enquiry may be one of his dominant occupations. The seeker after truth—the man of science, for example—may be actuated either by a love for truth as such, or by utilitarian motives, the hope of discoveries that may benefit himself or mankind. In the playful intelligence, on the one hand, and in intelligence as contributing to instinctive satisfactions on the other, it might seem easy to detect the two-fold basis on which these two types of intellectual disposition are built up. But though a playful origin may explain the adult's indulgence in intellectual pastimes (e.g. art, literature, chess, and even crossword puzzles), it will not account for the persistent seriousness of many truth-seekers.

The solution is here provided by the action of intelligence itself. For intelligence at the human level by its own exercise discloses to man its own utility. It teaches him firstly that it is by persistent truth-seeking that discoveries useful to man are made ; and again it reveals to him how much of human value results from truths sought and secured for discovery's sake. Hence the two types —the philanthropic and the disinterested truth-seeker. Though of course in any individual case both motives may be present.

Thus the disposition to the exercise of intelligence, claimed by some as itself instinctive, appears to be largely acquired through the recognition, made possible by intelligence, of the immeasurable value of its own activity. While we must also add that this acquirement (like all human acquirements) derives from an innate basis, namely, a capacity to apprehend relations, actuated by instincts on their own behalf, and thus tending to function as play in ' leisure ' intervals. But to assume a separate particular instinct of intelligence seems unwarranted and gratuitous.

From the position we have now reached it will be possible to attack with some hope of success the question whether intelligence is the servant or the master of the passions, the creature or the director of impulse. This constitutes the subject matter of the following chapter.

CHAPTER IX

INTELLIGENCE THE MASTER OF INSTINCT

To the psychologist who regards intelligence as an instrument or capacity, and not as a force, it might seem that the question whether intelligence is a servant or a master has already been answered. An instrument by definition implies some user, whose servant it is. But in speaking of intelligence as an instrument we are merely using a convenient physical analogy in order to expose one aspect of intelligence. Moreover, even if we regard it as an instrument it does not follow that instinct is its only master. We may avoid begging the question by putting it in another form : " Do I by virtue of my intelligence master or direct my impulses, or do I use it merely to satisfy them ? " This is the question which will now be considered.

Let us grant that we start life as creatures predominantly of impulse, that the infant, for the first year of life at any rate, is primarily occupied in obtaining satisfaction of physical cravings—he makes little discernible attempt to control them. We may further admit that animals lower than man throughout their lives show little (though perhaps some) evidence of rising above the level of instinctive satisfactions.

To the further question whether man in the course of individual development ever really rises above the instinctive level, and subjects his instinctive ' drives ' to the control of some higher authority the mechanist psychologist, where he is consistent with his premises, returns a negative asnwer. Moreover, it is surprising and significant that even so professedly anti-mechanist an author as McDougall appears to commit himself to a determinist doctrine. Indeed, on this very ground he has actually been charged with determinist inclinations. " Directly or indirectly," says McDougall, " the instincts are the prime movers of all human activity ; by the conative or impulsive force of some instinct (or of some habit derived from an instinct), every train of thought, however cold and passionless it may seem, is borne along towards its end, and every bodily activity is initiated and sustained. The instinctive impulses determine the ends of all activities and supply the driving power by which all mental activities are sustained ; and all the complex intellectual apparatus of the most highly developed mind is but a means towards these ends, is but the instrument by which these impulses seek their satisfactions, while pleasure and pain do but serve to guide them in their choice of means."[1] With authorities in both camps in agreement as to the subordination of intelligence (whether to instinct within or to environmental stimuli without) the counter argument seems badly off for support.

Let us turn now to common human experience, for it is human experience that supplies the data of psychology and which it is the business of psychology to systematize. As we all know, both our inner conscious experience and our outward conduct persistently contradict the psychologist's determinist conclusions. The parent and the teacher—and particularly the educated and enlightened parent and teacher—are alive to the duty of getting their children to practice self-control, the control, that is, of impulses instinctive or derived from the same. Enlightened self-control is accepted as an important (if not the most important) purpose of education. Moreover, our ordinary language (and therefore the thoughts it signifies) persistently carry the same implication. We praise and blame, respect and condemn ; award merit and demerit. Genuinely, and with meaning. But to admit differences of merit in a number of individuals all equally and solely dominated and determined by impulses over which they exercise

I

and can exercise no control, is a palpable absurdity ;
just as it is equally absurd on the same premise to
condemn or to punish a criminal, or to blame him for
degrading himself, or for making no effort to improve.
So far as we are determined by our impulses, we have
no further say in the matter ; and our so-called personal
goodness or badness is only a name for good or ill fortune.
If we go wrong, it is either our original impulses or our
environment that are at fault : the criminal would
seem to deserve sympathy rather than condemnation ;
while the virtuous man would deserve no praise for his
virtue. We engage, it seems, in practicing a perpetual
irony : an elaborately disguised untruth.

Lastly, let us turn to the most direct and most truly
intimate knowledge we possess—our own immediate
inner experience. Here, again, we find ourselves—and
again in proportion to our enlightenment and education
—repeatedly imposing checks upon our impulses ; and
aware of a conflict between impulse and some higher
authority. We are all aware, more or less, and more
or less often, of what we term the voice of conscience,
meaning by conscience, not a calculation of advantage
to ourselves in terms of impulse satisfactions, but a
claim irrespective of such calculation, and felt as
superior to it. This conscience claims our obedience in
spite of the instigations of impulse, or any desire to
secure our own pleasure. In daily life this struggle
between impulse and conscience is often over long
periods for many of us not keenly in evidence ; for
sometimes impulse and duty coincide, and sometimes
impulses are not so strong, nor the dictates of conscience
so clear and decisive, as to bring the struggle to a head,
or produce a vivid and impressive awareness of striving
on the side of conscience, or of yielding to a lower
authority. But in some moral crisis where we find
ourselves resisting a keen temptation we know, and
know intensely, that we are not engaged in balancing
conflicting satisfactions of impulse, but in inhibiting

impulse in the service of some ideal. The martyr at the stake, and the hero who prefers death to dishonour, is not merely calculating on the chances of an eternity of instinctive satisfactions, but is asserting some higher value, something not translatable in terms of instinctive satisfaction at all.

We may now briefly review two contrasting accounts of the nature of this over-ruling conscience, the conflict between which and impulse is a cardinal fact of human experience.

One view, adopted by the mechanist psychologist, is that the conflict is either a mere illusion, or, at least so far as the science of psychology is concerned, must be so regarded. Since, however, the systematization of mental processes and phenomena is the prime function of the science of psychology, that science has either to include all important classes of phenomena within its system, or, if it regards one class as negligible, to explain on what principle it justifies disregarding that class rather than any other. And again, if it regards that class as illusory, it has to offer some explanation why that class is there, how it has come to exist. It has to find a place in its system either for the phenomena themselves, or, if the phenomena be illusory, for the illusion. What purpose is served by this elaborate and ironical mockery ? Until some answer is forthcoming to this question, we may set aside the mechanistic assumption,* and accept, at least provisionally, the experience of conflict between principle and impulse as a real experience, real, that is, for a science of human psychology, which takes as its data the mental phenomena of man.

An alternative to the expedient of solving the problem by denying its existence or its relevance, is to admit the problem but attempt no solution. This is the attitude of those who regard this principle, this conscience, this

*The 'rationale' of this mechanistic viewpoint is considered in Chapter XIII.

higher authority, as something arbitrary, mysterious, unaccountable. In one case science claims defeat as victory, in the other it merely admits defeat. But, since the problem conceals the key to human character, it is necessary for a science of human nature to attempt its solution. It may help to clear the issue if we turn for a moment to two attempts recently made.

One of these is the hypothesis put forward by Professor Roback in his discussion of " Character and Inhibition " in the book entitled *Problems of Personality* written in honour of Professor Morton Prince.[2] Interpreting character as inhibition of impulse in accordance with a regulative principle he comes to the question why this inhibition should take place ; for in the last resort —as already pointed out above—it does take place in spite of any impulse that we can regard as instinctive or as derived from instinctive impulses. Now the man of character as Roback points out is distinguished by his superior consistency in adhering to principle irrespective of the impulse of the moment. In default of better explanation of this tendency to adhere to principle, Roback postulates the existence in each of us of an urge to consistency, which however varies in degree as between individuals.[3] Thus some attain more character than others. He suggests as physiological basis for this different resistance values of the synapses.[4]

His suggested explanation, however, merely leaves the matter where it stands. For since this urge is part of the endowment of the individual, it is tantamount to adding another to the number of the instincts, and to a reduction of character to the level from which he set out to raise it. On this hypothesis the moral conflict, the authority of conscience, the exercise of self-control, remain illusory, for Roback's " inhibition of impulse " is merely one hereditary urge proving stronger than another : we appear to be controlling our impulses, but really it is the stronger innate urge that wins. Thus Roback returns to the very position he has been contesting. On the other hand his "urge for consistency" contains a hint of an important truth.

A different solution is proposed by Professor McDougall. In his view the development of character consists in the building up of a system of sentiments or organized emotional attachments or attitudes towards ideas, ideals, or objects.[5]

Sentiments as they develop, may, however, conflict with one another. Harmony, or true unity of character, therefore demands the development of a master sentiment; and the only master sentiment capable of effecting complete harmony is the sentiment of self-regard. By this is meant a sentiment for the ideal or highest self.

The question then arises what is this ideal or highest self, this self above the self as socially accepted? What is this authority which may even claim to defy the social code?

To this question McDougall gives the answer that it is the self as viewed by an assumed ideal spectator.[6] But this merely shifts the problem on to the spectator; and surely many of us would add the comment that we are not conscious in moments of conflict of reference to any ideal spectator at all.

We must therefore make another attempt to face the problem. If we are only obeying another impulse, why the distinctive character of the conflict? For it is experienced not as a vacillation between rival impulses, but as a subjection and control of impulse by something experienced not as impulse, but as something higher, and—curiously enough, weaker—less instigating, but yet imperative. If, on the other hand, it is not another impulse, why are we impelled to obey it?

Before suggesting an answer to this question, we may observe in passing that to admit the reality of a separate or independent principle is to render one answer to the question which introduced this chapter, " Is intelligence the servant or master of instinctive impulse? " For intelligence on this hypothesis appears as servant not of instinct, but of this higher principle or authority, or rather as an instrument used by this authority in its control of impulse. But since of course none of us ever succeeds in securing perfect control of passion on all occasions, the degree to which intelligence thus dominates impulse varies from man to man, and from one occasion to another.

A corollary to this proposition is also worth noting. It is that the form of the question " Is intelligence the servant or master of impulse ? " makes a wrong assumption. It implies that the relation of master to servant is a natural law or a stable fact ; and that we are concerned with the ascertaining of a fact. The question would more fairly be stated : " Can intelligence rule impulse ? and, How far does it normally do so ? " The answer being that a higher principle, or, more accurately, ' you ' and ' I ' in virtue of a higher principle in us, can and in some degree do rule our impulses, and use our intelligence for the purpose. But we can return to the main question when we have carried the argument further.

So far then attempts to solve the mystery of this ruling principle have ended in failure. It still faces us as unaccountable and apparently arbitrary, at any rate it has not been exhibited as following any law consistent with its unique character.

The claim that we are now about to make is that psychology can consistently include this principle or authority within its system without weakening its position as a science, for the principle is not the arbitrary thing it appears to be, but observes a definite intelligible law.

The ideal (whether of self or spectator) for which the individual acquires or develops a sentiment is, it may be suggested, not an ideal derived from any mysterious or novel source, but one derived directly from intelligence itself. It is indeed the expression and outcome of intelligence. It is the result of intelligence apprehending the extended implications of the rules of social convenience. When the individual accepts from his fellows the social rule " Thou shalt not steal " he is enabled, by virtue of his intelligence, to apprehend the relations embodied in the rule, and to relate them again more widely. If taking what belongs to B is the act that is socially reprehensible, then for A to use B's ideas in a book he is about to publish, without acknowledgment, is equally reprehensible ; and so is maligning B, or taking away some valuable quality he possesses. So too is it wrong to tax the poor in order to relieve the rich (for this is the rich taking the property of the poor)—, or beguiling B into buying land at twice its real value ; and so on. By virtue of intelligence the individual apprehends the relations of similarity between varying situations, and thus extends the social rule and makes it more comprehensive. In virtue of his intelligence he apprehends the principle underlying the rule, the principle which it embodies ; and the sentiment which he has acquired for the rule becomes a sentiment for its underlying principle.

So long however as the extension of the principle, his apprehension of it in situations other than those to which it primarily applied, are extensions more or less acceptable to or accepted by his fellows, his adherence to the principle has social support, and he may be represented as acting from motives of personal convenience. In other words he does not, or need not, appear as rising above the level of impulse, or derived desires, for he may be obeying his law through social fear or the desire to excel or to be at one with his fellows—all these being motives which rest on an instinctive basis. But directly he apprehends extensions of the principle beyond those socially accepted, and even in opposition to the social code of his time, the explanation in terms of convenience no longer obtains. For he is found defying the social code or rule, acting not in fear of his fellows or from a

desire for their approval but in spite of his fears of them
and in spite of their disapproval.   The martyr accepts
the stake, and Socrates his hemlock.   The true nature
of that adherence to principle which constitutes the
highest type of character now becomes apparent.
The individual as an intelligent being *is vindicating the
authority of his own intelligence.*

And he has good reason for doing so.   For it is
precisely this intelligence itself which constitutes his
superiority over the insect and the ape.   In defying
its authority, he is defying and repudiating that which
he recognizes as his highest function and possession.
He is in fact degrading his highest self.   That self
however is not his highest self merely because it is so in
the eyes of an ideal spectator, but because it is the
intelligent self, the self recognizing its own highest
principle.   It is that principle which has, through
evolutionary epochs, been slowly attaining higher and
higher developments culminating in man.   For man to
disregard or defy its dictates is to repudiate that which
is the unique achievement of man.   It is that which
transcends instinct, and in virtue of which man's
behaviour can transcend and therefore control instinctive
behaviour.

Thus then the highest type of character, in which, as
McDougall puts it, the personality attains unity, is
achieved when character harmonizes with intelligence,
in other words when the principles to which the
individual adheres are the most comprehensive principles
which his intelligence can disclose to him.[7]   So far as
he adheres to these principles in conduct he remains
master of his impulses, and the victory is with him.   But
directly he yields to any impulse, where such concession
is not in accordance with these principles, he at once
experiences the discrepancy between what he recognizes
as his highest achievement and that which he shares
with the brute creation below him.   The man has
yielded to the beast.   Every such defeat therefore is a

blow to his self-respect, to his sentiment of regard for his highest self. Hence his shame, the emotion that accompanies not just defiance of a social code, but awareness of self-degradation.

If this account of the nature of the highest authority be the true one, an answer to the question of this chapter is now forthcoming. Intelligence is the servant of instinctive impulse so far and so long as it does not assert its own authority. The animal and the infant are at this stage. Man however happens to possess intelligence of such a level as to be able through it to universalize the principles underlying his social conduct.

So far as he approaches this universalization, and so far as he adheres to the comprehensive principles of conduct so derived, he brings, through intelligence, his instinctive (and acquired) impulses under control. Thus, on this further analysis, it appears that intelligence is not just the servant of the ideal, but is itself also the creator of the ideal. It is thus master in its own house. It sets up its own authority. The ideal is no mysterious arbitrary principle, or voice, or conscience, separate from and superior to intelligence, but is the very expression of intelligence itself ; the very embodiment of reason ;—the exact opposite of the capricious and the arbitrary.

We are now able to discover the element of truth in Roback's urge for consistency, and McDougall's sentiment of regard for the ideal spectator. It is of course consistency, and the most comprehensive consistency, which characterizes conduct directed by intelligence, for intelligence is the discoverer of consistencies in varying situations, and consequently harmonizes the behaviour that applies to them. But to describe it as prompted by an urge, and that urge a matter of endowment, nay further a function of a varying innate tendency to resistance in the synapses, is to reverse the truth. The man of character achieves consistency in spite of inconsistent innate urges, in spite of urges to inconsistency. Character he acquires not through following impulse, but through choosing to act consistently with his own highest self—his self as intelligent.

Hence also a certain appropriateness in the use of the phrase " the ideal spectator," as that for which he develops this regard, so long as we treat the phrase only as metaphor. For in its aloofness from the merely impulsive man (the slave of conflicting passions), in its calm detachment, intelligence may be. compared to a spectator. But the paradox must not be missed that in concrete fact the spectator is also in charge of the spectacle ; or, to put it more correctly, I as spectator, or I as intelligent, control myself as instinctive.

PART III

CHAPTER X

THE PROBLEM OF INTELLIGENCE AND VOLITION

It is one of the paradoxes of modern psychology that the student as he enters on the subject finds himself committed to a preliminary view of human nature, or a set of assumptions concerning it, the very opposite of those upon which all of us, including even psychologists, actually conduct our lives. In actual life we assume all along the line that man can and does initiate and choose his own behaviour, and is able to control and inhibit impulses he has inherited or acquired, and to act of his choice at the moment otherwise than those impulses prompt.

This is the premise implied in blame or praise, for when we praise or blame a fellow human being we commend him, not as we commend a machine if it is oiled and greased and working without a hitch, but as a being capable, in the act for which we praised him, of exercising an immediate control over his own activity and exercising that control in a certain (namely a right) direction. Conversely we blame him when he fails to exercise that control.

And on the same assumption does each individual blame or praise himself : blames himself for not having on some occasion acted otherwise than he did, or experiences a moment of pride or self-respect that in a moral crisis he chose to act in a way that he himself approved.

On precisely the same assumption does every teacher and parent educate his child to develop his character, meaning by character nothing more nor less than just the acquired disposition to control and inhibit impulse according to some principle or principles which he is to prefer, that is to choose in preference, to mere impulse. For if character is a fashioned will, it is the individual himself who is its fashioner.

But the modern student of the science of psychology finds himself as he goes on with his study becoming— often unwittingly and insidiously—indoctrinated with premises which directly contradict his experience, his unsophisticated experience, in life. This process of indoctrination is the more effective when as is usual it does not rely upon any professed discussion of these premises, but is implicit in the very nature of the student's occupation. He learns as it were by doing : he imbibes the doctrine because he begins by applying it. For since as a student of science he is engaged in seeking the laws, the uniformities, which underlie human behaviour, the assumption is that human behaviour can be expressed in uniformities, and that wherever he turns his attention they exist to be found, if only he searches diligently enough to discover them.

The doctrine thus quietly assumed by him has next to be defended ; for after all the discrepancy between the doctrine and the actual daily experience is, even in the present age with its scientific psychic dominant, too glaring to pass without notice. Persuasive arguments are easily forthcoming. They usually take one or other of two forms, or both together. On the one hand there is the argument that inasmuch as all science is in its nature a search for universal truths, it is bound to assume their existence, so that human nature as a subject of scientific study must be regarded as the expression of general laws or principles, and therefore as behaving in accordance with them. On no other assumption can science pursue its task.

The other argument is not always distinguished from the previous one. It consists in maintaining that the assumption which science makes about the universality of law is also true. Human nature must not only be assumed for the purposes of scientific study to behave in accordance with laws, but actually does behave in accordance with them, so that science is justified in its dogma.

It is to be noted that according to the first premise volition in the sense of an ability on the part of the individual to decide how he shall act in any given case disappears from the science of psychology ; according to the second premise it disappears from human behaviour itself. " All events are caused, that is, take place according to universal laws. An act of volition is an event. Therefore it is also caused. Therefore it does not cause itself. Hence the experience of volition as ourselves causing our own acts is illusory." This type of reasoning rests for its validity upon the second of the two premises : the assumption of the science of psychology is held to be true.

Most general discussions of psychology, particularly those issued as text books for young students, imply rather than assert the acceptance of both these dogmas, and by basing their whole exposition upon them insinuate them unresisted into the student mind, for to offer resistance to an influence we must first know it exists. Subject to the two psychic dominants of the period, the evolutionary dominant on the one hand and the scientific on the other, current expositions of psychology begin their treatment of the subject with those aspects of human behaviour which seem prior in time—its ' animal ' and physiological aspects—and again with those elements in behaving which are more readily expressible in terms of universal laws, the bodily mechanisms. Thus in current textbooks, or in more elaborate treatments of general psychology, we do not usually arrive at the topic of volition until the lower level aspects of human behaviour have been disposed of, if indeed we ever arrive at it at all. Coming to this unique phenomenon toward the end of his course, when he has already built up a scheme of behaviour which has no place for it, the student's temptation is seldom resisted to push the awkward intruder a little to one side, to refuse to recognize its true colours, to treat it as insignificant or as an impostor undeserving of a place in a 'science' of Psychology.[1] A few psychologists perhaps more honest or more perspicuous than the rest give it a glance of recognition for what it is—they face the problem momentarily (and more or perhaps less boldly), and pass (perhaps a little uncomfortably) to the conclusion of their subject.

Thus it comes about that a unique process in evidence in human behaviour, distinctive (at its highest level) of man, and therefore fundamental in any study of human as compared with animal psychology, a power in virtue of which man is capable of individual development far above that of the brute, is simply set aside. The problem is shelved, or outlawry pronounced against so irregular, so lawless, an intruder, who threatens to upset that universal harmony, to dislocate that huge machine, to the level of which it is the privilege of modern science to raise our human nature instead of leaving us to the random vagaries of a supposititious will.

There are, however, reasons to believe (1) that this treatment of volition in psychology rests on a false conception of the meaning and function of science; (2) that science has much to gain and nothing to fear by the frank admission on its merits of the authenticity of will; (3) that a systematic account of human nature is perfectly compatible with the admission of volition as a fundamental process; (4) that until it is given its due place in a science of psychology all that is most distinctively human in human behaviour goes unexplained.

In fine, on a proper understanding of volition an adequate and complete account of human behaviour depends.

It is convenient to approach these contentions by a preliminary consideration of variant interpretations of free will—the faculty of volition—and of the sense in which the term can most usefully be employed in human psychology. One sense of the term, ability to do anything, or to act just as one pleases, we may at once disregard. Man is so clearly limited in freedom of action, in freedom to do as he might wish, by his physical and social environment and by his own bodily constitution, and indeed by his mental limitations, that no one can seriously maintain the opposite.

We may consider three other interpretations. Of these the first is the view that within the limitations of the environment and of his bodily and mental structure man is free to choose and to set about undertaking any line or course of conduct irrespective of, and actually in defiance of, previous experiences or accumulated influence. By freedom of choice is here meant that his choice is determined by nothing other than the will itself ; the individual creates his own choice, initiates his own activity. It is truly spontaneous. He is his own cause.[2]

Free will in this sense too may be discounted. It involves discontinuity of behaviour. If at any moment we were capable of a completely fresh act, irrespective of anything in the past, our development would be chaotic and unpredictable. Indeed there would be no development at all. Moreover, there could also be no responsibility, for there would be no continuing individual to be responsible, or to be responsible to ; you of to-day are not continuous with you of to-morrow. You of yesterday have no necessary relevance to you of to-day. I cannot hold you at any time responsible for any act at any other time. Reward and punishment, praise and blame, encouragement and exhortation have no significance in a scheme of life that has no scheme, in which every moment of behaviour is a complete change from every other.

Moreover this extreme ' freedom ' is self-contradictory. It denies man freedom over himself, since he is no longer

K

master of his own future : his efforts to attain a goal,
to alter his own character or his environment, are
necessarily vain ; for the premise admits of no effective
resultant.   Complete momentary freedom is permanent
impotence.   We may therefore repudiate this conception
of freedom as self-annihilating as well as inconsistent
with our actual experience of ourselves.   It shares with
complete determinism the objection that it treats as
illusory the phenomena which it undertakes to explain.

Deserving of more attention is a third hypothesis, too
widely favoured by psychologists of professed determinist
and non-determinist schools to be discarded without
careful consideration.   The concept may be conveniently
approached by contrasting a man with a machine.   A
machine is not free to act, because its movements are
determined solely by the action upon it of the environment—an automobile does not start until the driver
starts the engine, and its movements, immediately or
originally, but completely, are under his control.   It can
do nothing of itself : it does not contain within it the
springs of its own activity.   It has no self-activity.
Man however is both machine and driver : he is self-
active ; the source of his movements is within.   He
is his own self-starter, and his own continuous control.
Thus his will may be considered as free from the sole
determination of the environment, for the individual
freely moves himself ; he is his own source of activity.

The argument however does not stop here.   For
after all, the will as chaos can also be so represented :
it also derives from within.   But, as contrasted with
the concept of the will as successive acts of caprice, the
hypothesis now being examined takes note of the
continuity and stability of the individual.   The will
is exhibited accordingly not as the momentary expression
of nothing in particular, but as the expression and
outcome of a self continuously developing from its past,
a resultant of its own past, and at any moment, so to
speak, the last word on the subject.   The will is thus

said to be free when it expresses the total personality.[3]
The will is free in that it is the whole man active, the
whole man expressing himself and not just the result
of the momentary action upon him of the environment.
So far as he expresses himself he is free, so far as he is
at the moment externally determined, he is not free.
Thus the term freedom is vindicated in that : (1) this
activity is determined from within, is therefore self-
determined ; (2) the self that determines it is the whole
self, not just the momentary or partial self. What
more freedom could be possible ? Here we have the
organism expressing its own nature.

Plausible as this theory appears at first sight it has
two fundamental objections for the psychologist
attempting to explain (that is to find a reasonable place
in his system for) the actual phenomena of human nature
and behaviour. In the first place it is just when the
man is not acting as a whole, just when the individual
is divided against himself, that the fact of will, the act
of volition, is most in evidence. And the second
objection is that the peculiar characteristics of the
experience of volition become on this account just as
illusory as on the most thorough-going determinism :
indeed the "whole man" theory may be only
determinism in disguise.

These two objections are not independent of one
another. Indeed the claim that the will represents the
whole man can be maintained only by regarding the
inner conflict as illusory. The man remains whole only
in so far as the conflict between the contending elements
within him is not regarded as a real disunion ; only,
that is to say, if we discount the volitional experience,
are we enabled to describe our action at any moment
as the resultant of our total past. On the whole man
hypothesis then freedom of the will is a misnomer.

W. B. Pillsbury may be cited as exemplifying this way
of thinking. In a chapter towards the end of his widely
used *Fundamentals of Psychology* he accords a brief

treatment to the subject of the will.[4] " All are agreed,"
he states, " that when the will acts, it acts in the light
of the motives : it is an expression of the nature of the
man ; and that in turn is dependent upon his instincts
and training, his immediate purposes and general
ideals." " Will is a term to designate the whole man
active, or a word used to distinguish between automatic
acts and those that imply choice and are controlled by
the system of purposes."

So far we may follow Pillsbury : he appears to be
admitting ideals and purposes as factors in the situation
independent of the instincts and man's innate attributes.
But if that were so, it is curious that in the body of his
book he has taken no trouble to explain how these
factors that control our behaviour arise and develop.
But it seems he does not credit purposes and ideals with
independent authority, so that he escapes this criticism
only however to encounter the other. For though a
man's acts " are the expression of the whole man and he
is free to do as he chooses " and " the man is free to do
what he desires " yet we are told immediately afterwards
" his desires are the outcome of his instincts and
environment and over these he has little control."

The will then according to Pillsbury is the whole man
active, and therefore free. But the man as he is at any
time is determined by his instincts and his environment
and therefore it is not free. For after all he is not
responsible for his instincts, and therefore not for his
environment unless something other than his instincts
determine his handling of it. But nothing other is
provided us. Thus the wholeness of the whole man is
preserved at the cost of his freedom.

Perhaps it was some sense of the inconsistency of this
conclusion that induced the insertion of the qualifying
' little.' Is it a grudging admission of the claims of
volition after all ? We are not told how this " little
control " is exercised. If volition as independent of the
instincts is intended, why does it receive no treatment

as a factor in psychology ?   If the man does exercise
any control at all, how is it that we get no account of
this important psychological interpolator ?   Pillsbury
appears to have slipped in a saving word at the last
moment in the interests of common sense.   But he has
sacrified his " whole man " in the process, for the man
exercising control over his instincts is no longer the
whole man : his instincts are on one side and something
else is on the other.   He is divided against himself.

What in Pillsbury is a momentary qualm appears
to be much more definitely felt by Woodworth.[5]   He
goes so far as to abandon the view that the willed act
represents the whole man.   But he is unwilling to leave
the whole man altogether out of the picture.   He
describes the volitional experience as follows :   " In
cases of conflict the lower motive being the stronger,
how can it ever be the higher motive gets the decision ?
Well, the fight is not just a conflict between these two.
Other motives are drawn into the fray, the whole man
is drawn in, and it is a question which side is the stronger.
Fear of ridicule or criticism, sense of duty, self respect,
ambition, ideals of self, concern for the welfare of another
person, loyalty to a social group, may be ranged on the
side of the weaker motive and give it an advantage
over the stronger."

Thus Woodworth contends not that the willed act
represents or expresses the whole man, but only that
it involves his activity—a very different proposition.
This proposition, it is worth noticing, is equally questionable :   for though it is no doubt true that in a case of
conflict or hesitation the individual entertains a number
of considerations, or is moved by a number of impulses
or emotional spurs, it does not in the least follow that
all the impulses or emotional incitements of which the
man is capable, nor indeed all that are relevant to the
problem, actually come in.   In the normal course of
associative memory a certain number of associated
experiences, and in the normal course of the functioning

of intelligence a certain number of fresh relations appear in consciousness, with their attendant emotions, but there is no guarantee, and indeed no likelihood, that the whole of the individual's emotional repertoire is repeated every time he considers a hard case. We know that it is not so. How often do we in looking back on a decision regret that some consideration and some very relevant emotion or motive failed on the occasion to put in its appearance, and we acted, as we think afterwards, wrongly.

There is of course no sharp dividing line between cases of conflict and cases of no conflict : there are all kinds of intermediate cases ; and there is no point at which the whole man suddenly begins to function—there are, as James has pointed out, all degrees between the act which is the outcome of a single strong impulse and the act which results from careful consideration,[6] where a variety of motives that do, or we think should, weigh with us are turned over in our minds, and we (not our motives—an all important distinction*) eventually turn the scale.

But what does Woodworth mean by the " whole man ? " He fails to define this term anywhere ; but that we are right in our interpretation of him his example witnesses, for he estimates his wholeness in terms of motives, fear of ridicule, sense of duty, concern for others, and so on. The fallacy lies in that frequent snare of the psychologist, the hypostatization of abstractions, as if a man were made up of a number of motives, as a house is of bricks. The wholeness of the individual is not to be estimated by aggregating the motives that actuate him in a period of conflict and hesitation, and claiming that if enough of them come up, the whole man has been drawn in.

There is yet another fallacy underlying the " whole man " argument—a fallacy which Woodworth's example brings out clearly. It is the assumption that an act

*This distinction is not, however, stressed by James.

is not a willed act unless it has been carefully considered, and a number of motives have been operative in deciding it. The degree of volition behind an act is not however proportioned to the amount of consideration or reflection preceding it, nor to the number or variety of the motives in play. I may strongly will an act from the single motive of altruistic sympathy. Or there may be operative only two conflicting motives, say love or tender feeling on the one side and fear on the other, as when a father rescues his child from fire in imminent danger of his own life. He may have been a timid man, and a strong effort of will have been required. But he certainly cannot be represented as the whole man active in the sense employed by Woodworth of a man, actuated by a number of motives and considerations, choosing his action as a consequence of all of them. The whole man is not in this sense drawn in. And, the point of importance here, the presence or absence of will in the act, or the degree of volition behind it, is in no way correlative to the " amount of wholeness " brought into activity.

Three conclusions follow from this examination of the " whole man " dogma. (1) Will is not the whole man active, in the sense ascribed by these and many other psychologists. (2) The presence or absence of will does not depend upon the presence of a greater or less number of an individual's range of operative motives. (3) It is just where the individual feels himself least whole, or where he feels himself divided against himself, that will most conspicuously comes in. It is being pulled in opposite directions, not being pulled in many directions, that provides one of the conditions (and note one, not the only, condition) in which will is likely to be most evident.

That this significant phenomenon of will is exhibited in just these cases seems too obvious and universal an experience to require dwelling upon. But the reader who still hankers after the view of will as the resultant of a set of instinctive impulses or motives might consider the following contrasted cases. Let him consider the case of a little child torn between the desire for the forbidden candy and the fear of punishment. The candy is near, the punishment distant and uncertain. He takes the candy. Another child, probably but not necessarily older, in the similar situation also experiences these conflicting motives. But he does not take the candy. Why? Because he has accepted a principle "No eating between meals," and eating the candy would conflict with this principle. In the first case the child may fairly be said to yield to the stronger of two motives. It should be noted that it is the active subject that yields, not one motive yielding to another, an unintelligible proposition.* Will is inconspicuous. But the second case is radically and fundamentally different. The child is not pulled between two motives, yielding to the stronger. *It is he who does the pulling. He, the human being, dominates both his motives. He is not pulled, at least not decisively pulled, by any motive, in the sense of an instinctive impulse at all.* He, the child, inhibits his motives by adhering to a principle. The child so inhibiting his motives† is ' willing.' His ability to do just this is his faculty of will. And in this respect we may fairly call him free. This ability constitutes his capacity for freedom. In the one case the subject imposes upon his impulses ; in the other his impulses impose upon him. Moreover, the subjective experiences are different. In the one there is an actual keen *consciousness of self-activity*, of initiative, of mastery (it is not possible to find an exact term for this unique experience) which is lacking in the other.

Anyone who interprets will as the expression of the whole man active, or as the resultant of an " ensemble

---

*The hypostatization fallacy again.
†The phrase " inhibiting his motives " is used advisedly, taking motive in the sense of impulse, whether innate or acquired (instinctive or habitual). The cardinal point is that I can oppose impulse, and will—at this level of its activity—is me doing so.

of impulses," as a recent textbook in psychology puts it, or of " the sum total of all our impulses towards activity ",[7] may do well to ponder these contrasting cases.

We may return to this or similar contrasts again, but it is pertinent now to point out that even if the whole man hypothesis is granted, it is misleading to call " the whole man active " free in any reasonable sense of the word. It does not follow that because an act may be claimed to express the whole man therefore the man is free. On the contrary there may be no difference in principle between this concept and complete determinism. The freedom claimed for it on the hypothesis is freedom from determination by the environment. The man acts in accordance with impulses from within, that is, from his own nature. But is this freedom real ? Is there any geniune choice of alternative acts ? If freedom from the immediate control by the environment is all that this freedom signifies, the freedom turns out to be illusory. For inasmuch as man's nature is on the hypothesis the outcome of and continuous with his past, and his past at any moment with previous conditions, his nature and behaviour are derived by direct continuity from his nature and tendencies at birth, and over them he had no control. His endowment was given him : he did not and was not free to choose it. Of two machines, one that is worked by hand and goes only so long as someone is working it, and another that, once set working, goes on, as we say, of its own accord, is there any sense in which one is freer to choose its own action than the other ? What freedom is added to an engine by putting all its works inside it ? Both are equally determined by the maker of the works. The one has no more genuine self-determination than the other.

But the freedom which you and I are conscious of when in a moral conflict we decide to choose the better and harder course is something more than mere awareness that the impulses moving us are within ; it is also an awareness that we—you and I—apart from the impulses that stir us, can and do choose the act, and proceed to execute it accordingly. It is not even true either that we decide the winning impulse or turn the scale in favour of one or other method. It is not the impulse that wins, but the decider. We may not be deciding *between* impulses at all. That is a false way of putting it. The case is not one of so many impulses present, with us as arbiters to choose between them. The experience is one of us, not our impulses, deciding the case. We will. We subject impulse to principle. Or, to put it still more precisely, I, aware of and accepting a principle, inhibit and control myself as impulsive. *I am not just impelled : I impel myself.* That I can do this constitutes my freedom.

Thus psychologists who rest satisfied with the whole man theory fail to explain this peculiar phenomenon. Nor have they any explanation of the *sense of freedom*, for they merely explain it away.* And on their theory of freedom the criminal is no more to be blamed for his crimes than the hero to be praised for his heroisms. For on that theory men act according to their natures, according no doubt to the whole of their natures, but according to something they cannot themselves help. Their natures were given them at birth, and a man's nature as it now is is nothing more nor less than a direct continuous outcome, by successive determinations by its own past self and the environment, of what was originally given him. The psychology of free will as merely " the whole man active " is inadequate to account for our intimate knowledge that we can help our actions, or if this knowledge is a delusion, for the existence or function of the delusion. And to present a will as free which you have already bound to its past is to throw dust in the eyes of the student.

Three accounts of the freedom of the will have now

*By resolving it into impulse, thus making the sense senseless.

been discarded as false, or inadequate for a science of psychology : (1) As the ability to do anything. A will unlimited. (2) As ability, within physical and physiological limits, to choose any action irrespective of one's own experience or development. An arbitrary causeless will. (3) As action in accordance with one's whole personality, as distinct from action determined by the momentary environment. A will determined by the total 'nature' of the subject.

There remains a fourth interpretation. This view, the one to be adopted here as the only view appropriate to a science of psychology, because the only view consistent with the data of psychology, may be summarized in the following propositions :

1. Man can and does exercise, in every conscious moment, a real choice of behaviour, that is to say, he is able to prefer and act upon some principle of behaviour other than momentary impulses given or determined from birth or directly derived therefrom.

2. In its clearest, most emphatic, and evolutionarily most advanced form this ability appears as ability to master impulse, that is to act in opposition to a felt strong impulse or desire and in observance of a principle or in pursuance of an end accepted by the subject as more desirable than the end to which he is impelled at the moment. This ability on this level of its exercise may be termed the freedom of the will. The individual may be termed free when and in so far as he exercises this freedom, that is, prefers principle to impulse.

3. Though, however, we may reserve the term free will for this its clearest manifestation, there is no sharp line at any point along a scale from the highest level of triumph over impulse (as of the martyr or the hero) down to the volition involved in an almost automatic act like that of rising from a chair, or suppressing a yawn. Indeed even action taken on behalf of impulse itself involves a certain level of will, that is of freedom to carry out the act or to do so in one way rather than in

another.   There is thus a sense in which our acts are
usually mixed, neither wholly free nor wholly determined.

4. The term freedom again may be used either of the
act or of a goal of attainment.   We may thus speak of
stages of increasing freedom, attained by acts of volition
in the past.   Free acts lead to a state or condition of
freedom.   Regarded as attainment man's will is never
completely free, but neither is it, so long as he lives,
ever completely determined.

5. The characteristic of volition is not conation but
initiative.   Consequently the level of volition of which
the individual is capable is limited by the level of his
intelligence.   Both phylogenetically and ontogenetically
the 'faculties' of intelligence and of volition develop
interdependently.

6. The freedom of the will is not, therefore, proportioned to the amount of effort entailed in carrying
out the 'intelligent' act, but to the extent to which the
act is determined by intelligence or by impulse.   It is
of course possible in a given case for the two to coincide.

7. According to this conception of the will, a free will
is not a will free to make any choice of action, nor a
freedom to act at haphazard within physical and
physiological limitations, but a freedom to prefer intelligent to impulsive behaviour.   And since intelligence
is the power of disclosing principles and laws, the will
is free so far as it substitutes adherence to principle
and law for a mere following of impulse.   This concept
of free will, be it noted, is in sharp contrast with the
concept, set up and knocked down by determinists, of
a will that is arbitrary and chaotic.   So far from being
chaotic it is a deliberate insistence upon principle, upon
law.   It is the preference of the rule of law over determination of behaviour by chaotic and random momentary
impulse.

8. This power of adhering to principle in defiance of
impulse renders the individual's behaviour to that extent
predictable, once we know the principles he has espoused.

But his behaviour is never completely predictable, even if we know all the external circumstances and his adopted principles of conduct, because he still remains free to adopt higher and more comprehensive principles as his intelligence reveals them ; and again because he may at any moment and on any occasion fail to exercise his freedom and be found following mere impulse instead.   (The phrase " mere impulse " includes not only the impulse of original instinct, but also that of acquired habit, for the impulse to act habitually is itself instinctive, or at any rate innate in all).

In actual fact of course even if the predictability of human behaviour be granted in principle, no one, not even his nearest and most familiar associates, ever attains, or ever can attain, a sufficiently precise and intimate knowledge of any individual's principles of conduct and at the same time of all the relevant circumstances on every occasion, to be able to predict with absolute certainty what he will do.   We could never in any case hope to predict with the same confidence as we predict the behaviour of the inorganic in, say, a chemical laboratory.

9. It follows then that so far as our knowledge of individuals is concerned the science of psychology can never hope to be an exact science, for human behaviour is in accordance with two inaccessible variants, one, volition, the other the contents and events in consciousness of the individual.   To neither of these has the outside observer the means of access, without the immediate co-operation of the individual under observation.   A science of psychology that aims at individual predictions is thus exceeding its powers : it is going beyond its terms of reference.   This of course does not mean that there is no room for a science of psychology ; it means only that it must approach its subject with a clear knowledge of its limitations and conditions.   It must adapt its methods and its objectives to the nature of its subject matter, and not begin its enterprise by

hastily transferring to the study of life methods and objectives which seem to serve (and because they serve) in the study of non-life. The generalization that what applies in the one field therefore applies in the other is a hasty and unscientific generalization.

10. But, as already pointed out, though volition makes human behaviour essentially unpredictable, it does not make it random. Nor does it mean that it is entirely free. The living being is capable of freedom in virtue of intelligence on the one hand and of volition on the other. Intelligence limits what he can do, what he will do depends upon volition. His freedom is thus limited by the degree of his intelligence. Intelligence is thus a limiting condition of will itself. After all no one can carry out a new act unless it first " comes into his head " ; and no one can act on a principle unless he is at least capable of understanding it. And some of us are more capable than others both of understanding and of discovering new principles of behaviour.

For this reason, namely his inferior intelligence, the ape's will is less free than the human's, and the worm's less free than the ape's. And where there is no intelligence there is no volition. The entrance of the one makes possible the exercise of the other.

In the last analysis, if volition in all its degrees were absent, intelligence itself could not begin to function. It requires some act or measure of attention. Even a dog turning its head towards the source of a sound is self-active, is exhibiting some measure of attention. Volition is present, though in a low degree. But it is no doubt conceivable that the level of volition at which we speak of the freedom of the will, the level at which we rise above impulse, might be absent without a corresponding absence of intelligence. But consider the futility of such a world. A world it would be of impotent dreamers, in which the genius would be he who dreamed the furthest and was most impotent and most aware of it. There would be no use for high intelligence in such a world ; and the science of psychology would be hard put to it to account for it in its system of behaviour. It would have no survival value. Then would be crucially tested the interest value of inert and useless knowledge. Is it true in the last analysis that mere knowledge, mere awareness of a truth, is in itself an adequate motive for pursuing it ? Unless this is so, intelligence would die of desuetude : it would not be worth while exercising it.

However that may be, in the actual course of evolution intelligence and volition have developed *pari passu*. That is to say, as we pass from level to level up the evolutionary scale, we find a higher degree both of intelligence and of volition at each stage. On the other hand, it is also true that within any stage the tendency is for volition to lag behind intelligence in individual behaviour. There are clear reasons for both these facts. As already pointed out, there cannot be a higher level of volition without a higher intelligence. Primarily, of course, it is limited by physical conditions. Neither dog nor man, for instance, is able, as a fly is able, to walk along the ceiling. But within our physical limitations our intelligence is a further limiting factor. A dog is perfectly able to make all the movements required in opening his kennel door, or fetching and arranging straw or leaves or cushions so as to provide himself a comfortable bed, or in closing his kennel door on a cold night to keep out the cold. But it takes a remarkably intelligent dog to do these things. His low degree of intelligence degrades his volition : it does not occur to him to do these acts. Far less is he able to plan and execute a new dwelling for himself, or a policy of mutual peace amongst the dogs of the neighbourhood, or to develop a system of signs like the human language. He may be physically capable of the movements involved in all these undertakings. But he does not, he cannot undertake them. Intelligence has limited volition. We cannot will what it does not occur to us to will.

But the second statement is also true. We often do not will what we can will. In animals this is evidenced in the lower level of volition where one impulse is at conflict with another ; for the animal is not, by reason of his limited intelligence, capable of volition subjecting impulse to principle. Of the several cats confined by Thorndike in cages, some made more effort to escape than others. We shall be told perhaps that some were more hungry. Perhaps, but they were not obliged to attempt to get out of their cages. A machine acts because it is obliged to : it has no say in the matter. But the cat initiates activity. The machine does not. Some of the cats showed more initiative than others. And some of them solved the problem sooner. They could because they would. Where there was a will,* there eventually appeared a way.

With man the same differences in volition appear on the same lowly level. For man ' comprehends ' levels of behaviour below him. But the higher levels of volition yield abundant examples. We make plans, plans for our own or the general welfare, but we do not carry them out. As a rule we must support volition with impulse. Thus many people do their best work if they are paid something for it. Impulse tips the balance. But the best work of all is work not done for money : here volition works on the highest level. In the one case intelligence was followed freely, in the other instinctive or derived impulse helped to determine action. And most of our actions are of this mixed nature. We act seldom quite freely. We may put the same thing another way by saying that volition of the lower is frequently exercised to support volition of a higher level. A lesser comes in to mediate a greater freedom. But so far as this is so, the will is the less free.

To summarize the main contentions of this chapter :

*I refer here to the lower level of volition, exhibited in impulsive behaviour.

As already claimed in the previous chapter the acts of every living creature are either impelled or intelligent ; impulse and intelligence cover the whole field. Most, perhaps all, our acts exhibit both these principles. But the two principles are not the same ; they are constantly conflicting. The power to act intelligently is volition, and the degree of volition expressed in any act is in direct ratio to the degree in which intelligence outweighs impulse. And just as intelligence rises from the lowliest to the highest levels as we come to man, so volition becomes increasingly volition : it becomes increasingly free. Thus man has much more free will than the lower animals. But in no sense is volition random or arbitrary ; for it is only so far as intelligence, the power of principle or order, participates, that volition participates also. All true initiative is intelligent, and volition is initiative. The freedom of the will is intelligence in exercise.

Only if we grant this conclusion can we understand the peculiar quality of the volitional consciousness, as most clearly exhibited in, say, a moral crisis. The peculiarity of the phenomenon lies in the very fact that while we feel ourselves impelled or drawn one way, we actually go another. This distinctive fact is completely missed if we regard the case as a conflict of impulses—a not infrequent way of expressing it. The case is one of impulse on the one side and something quite different from impulse on the other, namely the intelligent self. It is the self, the self initiative, the self imposing itself upon impulse, the self creating, the self a cause. The whole significance of human behaviour is completely missed, as modern psychology persistently misses it, by overlooking this simple truth : man can cause. Man can create his own motive, can move himself to action, in disregard of the motives supplied by impulse.*

* Also of course he can--and perhaps usually does—follow a ' given ' motive. So far as he does this, he fails to initiate : meliora video (intelligence), deteriora sequor (impulse)

Initiative is initiative : to act impulsively or habitually is not to initiate ; it is to act as one has acted before, either by original nature or by habit.

Until this truism has been accepted, accounts of the process of human development, and more narrowly of human (and also of animal) learning, are bound to fail ; they may account for the establishment or achievement but they cannot account for the first acquirement. No mechanical juggling with the conditioned reflex or with trials and errors can account for the introduction of a single new response. They give a more or less coherent account of the shifting or response within the original repertoire of instinctive or reflex or innately determined reactions, but they never account, and in the nature of the case cannot account, for the introduction of any response outside that original or innately determined repertoire. No amount of shifting or exchanging of ' bonds ' among the keys and the letters of my typewriter can introduce a new letter : the original list of responses remains the same, the only difference is that they are provoked by different (amongst the original set of) stimuli. And similarly no amount of shifting or exchanging can add or subtract from the original stimuli : all it can effect is to attach the old stimuli to different (amongst the original set of) responses.[8]

Until we recognize the co-operation of volition (the self initiating) with intelligence (the self apprehending the new—what it shall initiate) psychology will ' explain ' development in vain. It may juggle unintelligently with the two meanings of the word ' new ', confusing an old reaction new to that response with a genuinely new reaction, or it may dazzle us with a display of new patterns and designs without considering how they were created. The mechanistic psychology mistakes the beginning for the end, the Gestalt psychology the end for the beginning. For the question at issue is just the question how from original equipment is our behaviour shaped and fashioned ? One school answers by overlooking the curious shapeliness of the shape, the other by directing our attention to it and nothing else.

It is important in considernig volition to avoid mistaking it for conation, the experience of effort.[9]   Effort of course frequently follows the initiative act, but it is not therefore the same thing.   The overcoming of one's physical limitations is no easy matter.   And every innovation in physical movement or in conscious thought involves some new physical adjustment.   There is presumably some cerebral or some muscular modification. The accompanying affective tone betokens effort.   But the effort is not proportioned to the degree of volition. The ship-wrecked swimmer makes great efforts to reach the raft ; but his Volition* is at a low level, for he is acting primarily on a strong impulse.

Confusion over the relation of volition to conation is likely to deprive volition of its rightful place, and to land us back in a purely mechanistic psychology.   There is certainly a close relation between them, but they are not the same.   Moreover, they are not so closely related as to be proportional to one another.   All volition involves some degree of conation, but the degree which it involves depends not on the intensity or the level of the volition, but on purely physiological factors—habits of movement which have to be overcome, or a low degree of energy or a high degree of fatigue.   The horse under the lash of his driver, struggles his hardest to pull the load, and may even sink beneath it.   Conation is at a maximum ; volition is at a minimum, for his efforts are not the outcome of his own will.   He acts on impulse far more than on volition.   Similarly with the panic-stricken inmates fleeing from a house on fire.   Rather less intense is the conation of a game's player exerting himself to seize or throw the ball.   But his volition is on a higher level, though his conation is less.   A still

---

* In future, I shall distinguish Volition at its highest level (viz. independent of impulse) from volition or initiative at its lower level (viz. in pursuance of impulse) by spelling the former with a big V.

higher level of volition is shown by a student who sticks to his task in spite of his comrades calling him out to play. But conation is at a still lower intensity. The martyr who allows himself to be bound to the stake rather than recant wills strongly perhaps, but he conates scarcely at all. He may, of course, be extremely reluctant to be burned, but the measure of his reluctance is not the measure of his conation, it is the measure of his ' *unwillingness.*'

The identification of Volition with conation arises from confusing physical effort with psychical initiative. The difficulty of a difficult decision is not the difficulty of a difficult climb. The same word hides different experiences. The common factor is the presence of an obstacle with the experience of removing or overcoming it. But in the case of the decision the so-called effort which the volition entails is different in quality from the effort of toiling up a hill. The one is psychical, the other physiological. The one is reluctance or un-willingness, the other is physical stress and strain. The conditions which arouse them are different. A con-dition of the one is the anticipation of uncomfortable consequences ; of the other the presence of actual physical impediments or bodily fatigue or inertia, needing the greater strain to overcome them. In the case of volition no such difficulty may exist. Nothing prevents me from walking into the flames to rescue a burning infant : there is no physical inability to stop me. If I do not do it, it is because I am reluctant to do it ; I do not so will. Conation is proportioned to impediment, Volition to impulse. The experiences of overcoming an impediment and of mastering an impulse are different in quality. Volition is the active aspect of intelligence, the activity being the more pronounced as the impulses (instinctive or acquired) to be mastered are more insistent by original endowment or by habit. The self is felt more active in such a case. But in any concrete case Volition and conation are so inextricably mixed, as also are impulse and intelligence, that it requires clear introspective analysis to discriminate the two sets of factors. But the differences are psychologically of the highest significance.

The distinction between Volition and conation may be illustrated further from two not uncommon psychological types, the fanatic and the so-called strong-willed individual. The fanatic is a one-sided enthusiast who often lives at a high level of conation, but so far as his fanaticism is in question he does not display any high level of will. For his fanaticism is of the nature of impulse or of habit or more often of both combined. The out-and-out fundamentalist may be an individual who, as we may put it, has allowed himself to be carried away by an idea. He has signally failed to exercise control. He has refused or neglected to exercise his intelligence, or to be guided by its deliverances. Not initiative but lack of initiative is his characteristic. Volition is at a low level. And what are the impulses to which the fanatic has yielded ? Sometimes largely to the mere force of habit, but more often, for habit alone scarcely suffices to produce the fanatic, to the impulse of self assertion, of dominance, to the desire for power. He would impose his views on others, not as he wrongly rationalizes, because they are correct, but because they are his, the imposition of them upon others ministers to his pride. Some fanatics there are no doubt who appear as unselfish idealists. These illustrate the distinction more precisely. For, so far as they are true idealists, that is preach and practise in defiance of their stronger impulses and in obedience to the voice of intelligence, the term fanatic is a misnomer. As a term of opprobrium it ceases to apply. Rather it is the term applied to them by their more fanatical comrades by reason of *their* fanaticism—the familiar expedient of evading our weakeness by projecting them on to others. The true idealist is no fanatic in the sense of one who persists in a cause or an opinion in spite of its clear unreasonableness : he deliberately takes a reasonable view.   Of course it may happen that his opinion, though he has arrived at it after careful thought, may be wrong : it may be a less valuable opinion than that of even the majority of his fellows. He may be a very unintelligent or a very ill informed person, or both.   In that case he is exercising a high level of volition, the highest indeed of which he is capable, for no man can do more than prefer the intelligent to the impulsive action.   But the case must be extremely rare in which such a person would be regarded as a fanatic even by his fellows, for the reason that an individual of high principles (unmixed that is to say by self assertive impulses) is certain in his general conduct to display a considerateness and an altruism that will rob the judgment of his fellows of its sting.   They may call him a fanatic, but they will mean the less by it.

The concept of the so-called strong-willed person hides the same confusion between volition and conation. The strong-willed person is often in actual fact volitionally undeveloped.   There are in fact two types of strong will, one of which only is genuinely strong.   But the specious type sometimes passes for authentic, and is accorded an unmerited respect in consequence.   To the specious type belongs the individual who is in fact volitionally undeveloped, but happens to be endowed with unusually strong impulses of self-assertion and pugnacity.   His characteristic is aggressiveness—he is constantly imposing his ' will ' upon others.   He develops forceful habits.   But he is in no sense strong-willed in reality.   He is merely dominated by strong impulses ; to which he yields.   He learns no doubt to get his own way more often than his less aggressive fellows : getting one's own way is not so strong an impulse with them. Genuine strength of will shows itself quite otherwise. It is not concerned to get its own way at the moment, for it does not yield to the self assertive impulse.   On the contrary, the impulses of self assertion and pugnacity are under a strong control; the strength consists in the steady subjection of these as of other impulses to principle. The will is in evidence in the whole course of conduct, which is seldom marked, except on due occasion, by specially violent or forceful behaviour. Quiet equanimity of manner rather than impulsiveness marks this genuine control. The possession of the strong will is often not conspicuous at first sight. The strength becomes manifest with acquaintance. Nor does it follow that it wins so immediate or striking a ' success ' as its more impetuous opposite. On the other hand its influence is apt to be more lasting, for the simple reason that principle is that which lasts : it is the permanent behind the transient. The specious type exhibits conation with a minimum of Volition, but for the really strong willed conation is subordinate.

CHAPTER XI

FREE WILL AND A SCIENCE OF PSYCHOLOGY

WE can now attempt to substantiate the claims made in the last chapter that the failure to recognize the significance of Volition in psychology rests upon a misconception of the nature of science ; and that science has nothing to fear from a full recognition of the validity of Volition at its highest level.

Perhaps a practicable way of approaching this topic is to consider a number of common assumptions (not the less, indeed the more, potent in that they are implicit rather than explicit), which have come to impede scientific progress. It requires a science of psychology free from self-imposed restrictions to do justice to freedom in its subject—human behaviour. This chapter is an attempt to free it from some of these impediments. The assumptions are the following :

(1) That it is the business of science to get rid of mysteries.

(2) That science assumes the universality of laws in the sense of invariable uniformities ; and only on that assumption can science be pursued.

(3) That scientific explanation is necessarily mechanistic.

(4) That cause is either a kind of blind force or a term for the first of two in any uniform sequence of events.

(5) That the effect can contain nothing which was not contained in the cause.

It is proposed to deal with each of these fallacies or with the fallacies implied in each of these assumptions, in its relation to the question of the place of Volition in a science of psychology.

The Relation of Science to Mystery

In recent literature of psychological controversy it is not uncommon for one party in the controversy, hard up for an argument, to disparage his opponent as a mystic, a dealer in mysteries. The implication is that he is therefore not scientific—he has abandoned attempts at explanation by invoking the aid of some mystic force or entity. And there are writers on psychology, writers of considerable repute, who actually claim, as for example in explaining the thinking process, to have got rid of mystery—" It is as simple as playing tennis— there is no mystery about it."[1]

The fallacy that science abolishes mysteries is almost too naive and crude, one might have hoped, to demand serious exposure. Science has never abolished a single mystery, and never will. It has not reduced by one the number of mysteries which have presented themselves to the human mind. Explanation is not the withdrawal of mystery; it is only its more precise location. It may indeed be even maintained that the progress of science is marked by a multiplication of the mysteries that occur to us, not by a decrease in their number ; as the circle of scientific discovery widens there is room for more mysteries on its circumference. And at no time in the world's history have men been aware of more mysteries than to-day : we are all engaged in fathoming some of them. There are more not fewer discoveries awaiting us than ever before : and we are making them at increasing rate. Thus the mysteries appear not to be lessening within the modern period of the great advance of science.

Let us consider a simple instance. Is there anyone of us who really believes that we can ever understand why the impinging of etheric vibrations (or their modern equivalent) of a certain number and rate upon the retina should result in that particular quality of consciousness we call red ? We may discover the physical conditions of the event called red, but can we ever hope to explain the event ?   It remains a mystery in the sense that it cannot be resolved into any experience simpler and more familiar than itself.   Just as little can we hope to explain, in the sense of removing the mystery from, any single event in consciousness—and to us all events are events in consciousness (though they may be events outside consciousness as well)—nor the mysterious fact of consciousness itself.   That the human mind is constitutionally incapable of removing mysteries even in the most familiar and ordinary events is a truism which escapes notice only because it is so familiar.   For we are all apt to overlook the obvious.[2]

The writer who maintains that there is no mystery about thinking because it is as simple as playing tennis himself overlooks this simple truism.   For playing tennis is a very mysterious process, just as mysterious as thinking is.   To convert thinking into terms of tennis playing, even if he succeeds in doing so, is not to get rid of the mystery of thinking.   It is merely to render one mystery in terms of another.

To charge an opponent with mysticism, in the sense of a belief in mysteries, is thus in effect to convict oneself. It is to claim a supernatural because a superhuman intellectual power : the power of getting rid of mysteries.

What science does attempt to get rid of is not mystery, it is magic.   The plausibility of the anti-mystic argument rests upon confusing the two.   Science attempts to discover certain connections, or relations, which appear, so far as we are concerned, to hold invariably between certain phenomena ; to establish certain uniformities of nature.   These discoveries are made by means accessible to all and result from the exercise of the ordinary human intelligence.   The assumption of the possession by individuals of peculiar powers and of their access to processes inaccessible to the ordinary human intelligence working in its normal way is the characteristic of magic.   If there are any psychologists who really do believe in magic, they merit accusation and exposure accordingly. But to charge with mysticism or a belief in magic potencies psychologists who do not accept these doctrines is to confess oneself balked for better arguments. It is the resource of the impotent.

To consider the bearing of this upon Volition. It is not the duty of science to reject Volition on the ground that it introduces a mystery. For science multiplies mysteries, it does not abolish them. It is the duty of science to reject Volition from the scope of the science of psychology if Volition implies a magic potency, that is, the possession of any peculiar power in individuals and their access to processes generally inaccessible. But to admit the existence of Volition is not to admit magic. For Volition is the property of all men, not the peculiar property of an individual : and the process of willing is open to investigation by us all. Volition, like consciousness, or red, or sound, or the experience of pleasure or pain, is a mystery, but it holds no magic. It is itself one of the interesting uniformities of human nature, and it exhibits in its functioning certain interesting uniformities. It is therefore the duty of science not to reject it but to discover what these uniformities may be. The taboo of Volition on the ground that it is mysterious is then the first impediment from which science can free itself.

The Relation of Volition to Law

A second assumption is that since science assumes and is bound to assume the universality of law, therefore the science of psychology can not recognize Volition as genuine initiative since this would interfere with the reign of law.

The immediate answer to this argument is that science is primarily interested in the search for truth, and therefore does not begin its search by assuming at the outset the particular form which that truth will take. For to do so is to beg the question. Science therefore makes no such preliminary assumption as that the universe, or man as one of its phenomena, is completely comprehensible in terms of invariable uniformities, or that man's whole behaviour is the outcome of universal laws. To make that assumption without adducing proof is to prejudge the verdict.

Science begins by taking its data as it finds them, and to this the science of psychology is no exception. Amongst one of its most interesting data, especially in the case of man, are the unique phenomena of Volition ; which group of phenomena science considers on their merits, unprejudiced by preconceptions or assumptions taken over from some school of philosophic speculations. That many men of science are unable to take this attitude indicates the difficulty of scientific detachment, the difficulty of prosecuting science in a scientific spirit. To science every experience is equal.

But to many this answer may not seem to get rid of their difficulties. Science, they will say or feel, is in practice bound to assume law, for otherwise how can it rely on the universality of any of its generalizations ? A generalization is a generalization, a statement of what holds universally. It is impossible for science to carry on its work if we admit that generalizations may not obtain. Is science to lose faith in herself ? To go on pursuing a futile quest for generalizations that do not exist ? This argument, however, assumes a needlessly extreme position. Whether in the long run, or in the last analysis, there is no compromise, no intermediate position, between universal universality and an ultimate initiative is a question not for the scientist but for the metaphysician, whose business it is to examine the products of the sciences if by chance he may discover a workable synthesis. So far as the scientific investigator of human behaviour is concerned, he is met by the simple fact that an assumption of universalities in one sphere of phenomena (the physical sphere, the sphere of the inorganic) and of initiative on the other (where life comes in) is actually found, so far as our daily experiences and conduct go, to be a perfectly working compromise, indeed the only workable plan we are aware of.

If on the one hand there were no uniformity at all, we could not carry on our lives for a moment, for we could not rely on anything being where it was or happening as it did on any previous occasion. We could not indeed continue to live. But on the other hand if there were no initiative, we could not even begin to live at all— there would be no life, nothing that we could dignify by the name of behaviour. There would indeed be nothing to behave. For mere uniformity is the negation of activity of any kind. For movement, activity, is *ipso facto* the upsetting of the *status quo*. It is initiation.

But whether the reader is prepared to accept the last statement or not, at any rate, and this is all that need be admitted for the scientist, we do actually work the compromise. Pragmatically, it works. We are exercising initiative in taking advantage of the uniformities of physical, and so far as they obtain, of human nature every moment of our lives. Just this is human behaviour. A scientific study of human behaviour is partial and inadequate which considers one side of it and not the other. The business of science is not to consider only the uniformities, but to investigate the compromise. It is just here that the peculiar interest of the scientific study of human behaviour comes in. It lies in discovering, to put it paradoxically, the uniformities, the laws, which condition the compromise.

Thus the business of the scientist, the disinterested student of human nature and behaviour, is not to degrade man as a machine nor to enthrone him as creator, but to be ever disclosing the relations between the two. If all creator, then there are no laws to investigate—we move in a region of magic. But if all mechanical—there is no man left to investigate. There remains the fascinating problem of the interconnections between the two.

This is the sphere of the science of psychology. The laws of these interconnections await discovery. But they may be only contingent laws. Moreover, they admit of degrees of regularity. There are many laws which hold for instance so long as we continue to will alike. The laws of human behaviour are thus both laws contingent and laws conditioned. If I perceive, there are certain uniformities of conscious process. But I may not perceive. The laws of perception are contingent laws. The average death age of a certain population is, say, forty-five years, and the average expectation of life at forty-five for that population is twelve years. On this basis insurance companies may determine their premium rates. And with fair confidence. But this law is also conditional; for human initiative taking advantage of other laws may alter the average. We may start living more healthy lives. Even our average stature is to some degree conditional on our own initiative. The average stature of women in England has risen noticeably in recent years. They have taken to outdoor pursuits, and more rational living. Both contingent and conditional laws are involved here. A contingent process is one that happens uniformly, if it happens. It is conditional when the process itself is more or less alterable at our Volition.

Hence there is no justification for the claim that science can be usefully and fruitfully pursued only on the assumption that all the data are reducible to invariable uniformities. Her business is not so to reduce them but to find and formulate the invariables within the variable.

The View that Scientific Explanation is Necessarily Mechanistic

The plausibility of this belief lies in overlooking its equivocal meaning. If all that is meant is that it is the business of science to disclose uniformities or mechanisms, and if we reserve the term explanation for these disclosures, the statement is unexceptionable. The fallacy lies in taking the statement to imply that since scientific discovery is the discovery of uniformities, therefore there is nothing else to discover, or rather there is nothing else existent. Or, to put the same thing another way, it lies in the assumption that whatever is is uniform, and is thus open, at least in principle, to expression as a uniformity. All human behaviour, and perhaps all phenomena,[3] exhibit at the same time both uniformity and non-uniformity. Volition is itself an example par excellence of this combination. As a characteristic of human behaviour it is itself a uniformity; that is to say, it is the common, the uniform, property of man. Moreover, it is also uniform in its procedure, and has uniform limitations. It works uniformly in only one direction, namely in that indicated by intelligence, or by a relative degree of intelligence. All human behaviour is uniformly either impulsive or volitional, either impelled, or guided by intelligence. From this law there is no escape. And from the law of free volition, that it operates in the more intelligent and less impulsive direction, there is no escape. So much for its mechanism. So much can science fruitfully disclose to us.

But we are not justified in concluding that the story of volition ends just here. On the contrary we know it does not. For there is left the question on what occasions do we will and on what do we follow impulse. And on this science can do no more than describe the occasions after they have happened. She cannot predict. She does not and cannot know the answer. Indeed no one knows, not, till he wills his act, the doer himself. If he did, he would prejudge his own volition. Again, he may mean to will, but fail to do so. He may, that is to say, initiate the thought, but not the action.

Thus scientific explanation deals with the mechanisms of will satisfactorily enough, and usefully. But the

explanation of will, in the sense of the complete*
explanation of it, is not therefore mechanistic. There
is something beyond the scope of scientific explanation.
All that science does is to discover some things about
the way it works. We are therefore not entitled to
conclude that because science discloses the mechanisms
of activity and of behaviour, therefore it can recognize
only subject matter or events which are completely
mechanical. Nor conversely may we conclude that
because human behaviour exhibits volition therefore
much of it is not susceptible to scientific explanation.
There is also the uniform.

If that be so we are free from the impediment which
those set up for themselves who hold that because
explanation is mechanistic, therefore science can treat
human nature only by denying to it all that is non-
mechanistic. Rather is it concerned to examine and
reveal the mechanisms involved in the procedures of
the non-mechanical, and in so doing to give its due
place to the non-mechanical as well as to the mechanical.
It goes beyond its province when it assumes as its initial
dogma that its function is to render one completely in
terms of the other, or to ignore the existence of either
of them.

In point of fact scientific explanation never succeeds
in reducing a single event that it investigates to
mechanism *and nothing else*. There is always something
left unexplained. We may investigate the behaviour
of the atom or the electron, but there is still the atom
or the electron left. We may investigate the conscious
processes, sensation, perception, attention, and so forth,
but there is still consciousness unexplained. We may
investigate the conditions and limitations of Volition,
but Volition itself remains outside the reach of science.
But of course this does not mean that science is to
refuse to recognize its place, any more than it refuses

* *i. e.* the resolution of it into something more familiar and self-
evident than itself.

to recognize the place of sensation, perception, or consciousness in the concrete events which constitute human behaviour. We can give no coherent account of human behaviour or human development by leaving them out.

Inadequate Concepts of Cause

The term cause has tended to pass out of fashion in modern science, at least where the writer is aiming at precision of statement. In a certain sense it might be held that there are no causes. Modern science is more concerned to discover uniformities than to disclose causes. The term is becoming discredited, because it involves an unwarranted personification or anthropomorphization. The term 'maker' or 'determiner' is reading into the facts more than we find there. All we find are uniform processes, invariable successions; and we are not justified in adding to the former of two events which happen in succession a kind of power over the other, making it occur. There is no series of powers passing in succession along the causal series endowing each effect with some initiative in turn, whereby it causes or makes happen the next event.[6] No such potency is discoverable. To read that into them is to endow them with the attributes of the human will : it is an unwarranted humanizing of the non-human.

On this ground the term *cause* is mistrusted in science, as carrying some implication beyond that of mere uniformity of occurrences. And frequently nothing is put in its place, no explanation of these uniform occurrences is forthcoming. Science is concerned, on this view, merely with describing what happens, with disclosing the uniformities. Further than this it is not the business of any particular science to go.

So far as concerns physical phenomena this attitude of modern science[7] may or may not be justified. But it does not follow that because the notion of cause as a kind of inanimate force making things happen has been

M

ruled out of physical science therefore there is no place for cause of any kind in any part of experience. It has been noted that the idea of cause as a determinant of movement or activity was taken over into physical from psychical phenomena. This transference may have been illegitimate. But it was possible to take it over only because it was already an actual human or psychical experience. We are constantly aware of ourselves initiating behaviour ; and in this sense, the sense of immediate initiators we experience ourselves as causes. We have no other direct experience of cause at all, and from no other source can we derive our notion of cause as maker. Apart from this unique experience the concept of cause as blind *force* itself could never have occurred to us. And inasmuch as the only experience of cause we possess is that of ourselves, intelligent conscious beings, initiating action, the burden of proving that a *blind* force ever exists or can exist lies upon those who make use of that concept. There is no evidence that it does exist : the only causes we know are of a different kind—living beings. To ascribe causation to non-life is to go beyond our direct experience ; and so far as investigation has gone beyond the available evidence. The only scientific attitude then is to admit as a datum of science the ordinary human experience of causation, but to make no use of cause in any other sense, until there are good reasons for so doing. To do so is a priori dogmatism : directly opposed to the whole spirit of science. The only initiators then that we are aware of in our immediate experience are living beings— ourselves.

Moreover there is an important implication in this experience of cause as initiator. It involves a repudiation of the assumption that there can be nothing more in the effect than there was already in the cause, the facile assumption of science in the nineteenth century,[8] which has so unfortunately influenced psychology in the twentieth.

There is no reason, however, to assume it valid. The absolute equation of cause and effect is an assumption which may or may not be found to work in the physical realm, but certainly we are not warranted in therefore assuming it of the psychical. About the learning process —to take an example—the significant and truly interesting thing is not its conservation of the old, but its initiation of the new. Indeed the very fact of cause itself implies an introduction of the new : you cannot initiate the old—repetition is not initiation. It is this very power to introduce the new that characterizes intelligence and volition. Intelligence is a new revelation, volition a new creation. One is the new in awareness, the other the new in act. All human development hangs thereon. Uniqueness is a measure of the degree to which intelligence and volition are what they are. Take away the new and they vanish with it.

The statement that the effect can contain nothing that was not in the cause really implies a mistaken analogy. For the form of the statement, the use of the word ' contains ' assumes a material occurrence. The analogy between cause and effect, on the one hand, and a vehicle and that which it contains, on the other, is a false analogy. There is no doubt a material side to all acts of causation : all causes use matter as their instruments. And the amount of matter, or energy or whatever term is used to express the fundamental material fact, is perhaps neither increased nor lessened by any act of causation. The measurable remains measurable. But cause makes no such claim on its behalf as that it alters the total sum of matter. Its newness is newness of another kind.

The statement that the effect contains nothing that was not in the cause merely implies an identity of *ingredients*. The material concerned is in both cases the same. But to admit this point (though ultimately the point may prove baseless) is not to admit that the

effect is in no sense new.   One thing new is the arrangement, the form, the inter-relations, of the material.
And after all, if matter is all reducible to electron-protons
or some simple identities or entities of uniform character,
rearrangements are all that is possible.   All originality
is rearrangement.[9]   In this sense the effect may be
importantly different from the cause ; the re-combina-
tions of elements or units may make all the difference
in practice.

If this holds, as we must admit it does in the physical
world, what reason is there for denying it of the psychical
world ?   For   we   experience   these   changes   just   as
immediately.   The firing of a gun may result in very
important re-arrangements of matter, so may the creation
of a cake or a chemical compound.   And these re-
arrangements may and do have very different appearances
and very different effects.   In other words the effect is
not just a re-arrangement, except as concerns the
material constituents.   The re-arrangement itself is not
the effect ; the effect is the practical resultant of the
re-arrangements.   This, not the ultimate units, if there
are any, constitute the new, are the essence of the
effect.

To hold then that the effect contains nothing that
was not in the cause is either fatuous or fallacious.   If
it means merely that the ultimate units of matter are
always the same, we may grant the point (at least
provisionally) while noting its non-significance.   If it
implies that the re-arrangements of these same units
are only re-arrangements, and *therefore nothing new*, we
reply that it is just on these re-arrangements that the
newness of the effects depends.   The effect is the
resultant of these very re-arrangements.   And it is
different from its precedent cause, often very significantly
different.   There is something completely new about it.
The one thing that the re-arrangement is not is a *mere*
re-arrangement.   New relations have been set up
between the constituent units, and these new relations

constitute the newness and give rise to further new relations—the ostensible effect. In other words the realities of our practical life are or may be just these very new differences in relations—the elements or units or atoms or whatever we name them being non-significant.

If this is so on the physical level why deny it equally of the psychical, for experience yields the same data to psychology. The experience is indeed more direct and intimate. We are repeatedly doing new deeds and thinking new thoughts. What point is served in denying their newness on the ground that a meticulous analysis of such constituents as are accessible to analysis discovers only old constituents? Such a contention is beside the point. Shakespeare was not the less original because he used ink and pen and paper, and wrote in words which were already in the dictionary, or because he used arm and hand and finger when creating Hamlet. He yet discovered the new. He created. But we do not need to select Shakespeare, or cite the unusual, for evidence of the original. Everyone of us every day is making more or less practically important re-arrangements of the old, re-arrangements in which the effect is not the mere fact of re-arrangement, but the new resultant of the re-arrangement. Not the re-arrangement but the new inter-relations it sets up. We study new books, we come to new conclusions, we wear new clothes, we try new diets, we are never quite the same even in our accustomed movements and performances; and some of these re-arrangements mean very different effects. We are in fact constantly introducing the new. The effects are very different from their causes.

The truth would be better put by saying that the effects are very different because of their causes; for the argument we are combating depends for its plausibility on a particular notion of cause. It regards a cause as a state of matter preceding another and different state of matter, to be called its effect But this is to deprive the term of its value. It is to regard the whole course of the universe as a series of states of matter just happening one after the other with nothing to mediate the changes. The term cause in its proper use is just this mediator of the changes. We are immediately aware of this mediator in ourselves, and we assume some mediator for the changes in the physical world, for we have no other way of comprehending them. Once we admit that the changes in the physical world are not uncaused, that they have causes, and once we admit that these causes are mediators or initiators of the changes, what right has science which implies cause in the inorganic to deny initiation in the organic ? So that on that score Volition (cause in human experience) is not only permissible but actually in consonance with scientific assumptions themselves.

Summarily then we may venture the following suggestions about cause and the relation of cause to volition :

(1) The notion of cause as a blind force rests on an unwarranted transference to the field of physical phenomena of a concept derived from the field of conscious experience, and may be dismissed.

(2) It does not however follow that the concept of cause should be discarded from the field in which cause is actually experienced and from which the notion is derived. It would be as unscientific to dismiss it from a field in which it obtains as to retain it in one in which it does not. In the one it is, in the other it is not, a *directly experienced* experience.

(3) In the field of conscious experience cause figures as Volition ; of cause in no other sense are we *directly conscious*.

(4) Hence it is in accordance with the spirit and principles of science to admit cause in this sense as a datum of the science of psychology.

(5) The identification of cause with effect, or the notion that there can be nothing in the effect which was not in the cause, does not apply to the concept of cause

and effect in the sense in which they are appropriate in psychology. They may or may not apply to cause in the set of a state of material units or factors and effect as another set successive in time to the previous set. But to cause in the sense of that which mediates a change or re-arrangement of matter and to effect in the sense of a new set of relations between material units so re-arranged the assumption does not apply. The effect in the sense now intended is essentially new and new not in spite of but owing to the cause.

There is then no warrant for excluding the notion of cause as thus understood from scientific psychology.

CHAPTER XII

IS VOLITION UNIQUE?

THERE is no more severe test of the scientific spirit than willingness or capacity to throw one's acquired and habitual preconceptions aside and to approach one's subject *freely*. Particularly difficult, as also particularly needful, is it to avoid subjection to the psychic dominants of the age ; but ability to do just this is the crucial test of a scientific attitude. One of the period's dominants is a preconception as to the meaning, the true conno-tation, of the term science itself ; and in consequence a prejudiced conception of the science of psychology. Now the difficulty in dealing with misleading psychic dominants is that they unwittingly, gradually and insidiously, and therefore mostly unresisted, secure their hold—they creep upon us from all sides unawares and in all sorts of disguises, so that we find that we have already accepted them as friends, often in our intellectual immaturity, before we have a fair chance of discerning their true character.[1]

Since it is the object of this discussion to claim and vindicate the need of a radical change in our concept of a ' science ' of psychology, and to free ourselves from a current psychic domination, no excuse is required for devoting another chapter to the meeting of actual and anticipated objections to the arguments advanced on behalf of a new (though also a very old) point of view. Yet I claim no originality, for all that is being attempted is the reconciliation of psychology with actual experience. The originality if any consists in not attempting to be original, in resting content with the eternal truths.

In the hope then of clarifying the principles so far propounded it may be helpful to consider a number of specific criticisms to which my inadequate exposition has, or may have, given rise.   They may be summarized as follows :

(1) A unique faculty of Will or Volition has been invented which is gratuitous, and unilluminative.

(2) This involves the fallacy of hypostatization.

(3) Will in its own rights involves a peculiar power to *intervene in natural processes* and thus offends against the reasonable sentiment for a law-abiding universe.

(4) The term Will is used inconsistently, being regarded as now in opposition, now in obedience to impulse.   Initiative and uninitiative.   It cannot be both.

(5) Moral distinctions are inappropriately introduced, specifically in the use of the terms higher and lower for different types of behaviour.   These are better omitted from a *psychological* discussion.

(6) Volition is not necessarily an illusion because, or if, it merely expresses natural laws, or is taken to be subject to determinations.   Hence the mechanist need not be called upon to explain an illusion he need not admit.

(7) The martyr and the hero are unfortunate examples to take of Willed behaviour ; why not take a big financier or a ' Butter and Eggs ' man ?

I shall begin by dealing with the first objection, confident that the rest will fall into place as we go along.

(1) *The Sense in which Volition is Unique*

Of course all acts of volition are in one sense unique, just as all events are.   No event ever happens twice—another event may happen very much like it.   There is no such thing as an actual recurrence.   But as no one is likely to maintain the contrary, we may dismiss this kind of uniqueness as not intended by the objection.

The term may be applied to volition in three other senses ; it may be meant by unique :

a. That volition is being regarded in this treatise as

peculiar to man, that man has somehow been empowered
with a special power or faculty not found in the brute.
And no satisfactory case has been made out for this
breach of continuity.

b. That whether we confine volition to man or not,
yet it is being conceived as something other than,
additional to, superimposed upon, evolutionarily preceding phenomena.   There is no warrant for such a
doctrine of discontinuity or of ' epigenesis.'

c. That volition is conceived as a special and peculiar
property of mind distinct, and set apart, from other
ordinarily recognized mental processes and phenomena—
perception, memory, imagination, impulse, etc.   There
is no reason for thus isolating it.

To consider these interpretations in turn.

*a. Is volition unique in the sense of being peculiar to
man ?*

The answer to this question should present no
difficulty.   A high degree of Volition is peculiar to man ;
a low degree is also exhibited in animals next below man
in the evolutionary scale ; and for the matter of that
some degree (however low) obtains wherever there is
life.   But if we prefer to reserve the term Volition for
the exercise of only the highest degree, then we can
claim Volition as peculiar to man ; man, we can say, is
the volitional animal just as we can claim that man is the
intelligent animal by reserving the term intelligence
for the highest degree of its exercise.   More correctly
we may say that man is *peculiarly volitional*, just as he
is peculiarly intelligent and peculiarly susceptible to
humour and peculiarly imaginative.

Volition is important in human psychology because
it bulks so importantly in human behaviour, not because
it is there for the first time in evidence, certainly not
because it has no lower stages of development in lower
stages of animal life.   No such discontinuity, no such
' peculiarity ' is implied.

But in the form of inhibition of impulse or

subordination of it to a principle consciously entertained
and determined by the individual himself Volition is not
found at levels of behaviour below man, and may thus
at that level be claimed as peculiar to him. This does
not mean that there is no genetic continuity between
Volition at this highest level and the level of self activity
reached by a dog forsaking its bone at the call of its
master or between that again and the first symptoms
of spontaneous self direction exhibited by the lowly
stentor rejecting the offensive carmine particles after
frequently accepting them.

  b. Is Volition an additional faculty ?

We are now provided with an answer to the criticism
that volition is regarded as implying a sort of ' epigenesis,'
a something super-imposed upon evolutionarily previous
phenomena. In the sense that Volition of the highest
degree involves the addition from some special source
of a separate power discontinuous with what went before
the criticism is clearly unwarranted ; for no such claim
is advanced, nothing more is claimed than is claimed
in every case of evolutionary development, namely
that development itself has taken place, there has been
some form of successive change. From the stage of
direct execution of impulse to the higher stage of delayed
(or partially inhibited) execution of impulse, to the still
higher stage of completely inhibited impulse, there is
no sudden leap—there has been no sudden imposing
of will upon a stage where no will was. Successive
change, evolution, development, characterize all
phenomena ; so that there is no reason for repudiating
will on the score that at some stage in the past it was
less in evidence than it is to-day. And development
after all is implied by all comparative psychologists,
for it is the obvious observable fact which they set out
to explain. Will then, since it involves no epigenesis,
cannot be rejected on that count.

  c. Is Volition a peculiar and distinct mental property ?

Thirdly, the difficulty about the uniqueness of volition

may arise from the suspicion that some extra faculty or function as it were is being introduced, other than the customarily accepted aspects or functions of mental activity, sensation, perception, memory, imagination, emotion, conation, impulse and so on.

The suspicion that a separate faculty or function has been somehow added will be removed by disentangling the relations between volition and these various psychological concepts, for it can only arise by confusing different kinds of concept.

Volition is not to be regarded on a par with sensation or perception or memory or imagination, as an assumed addition to them, but is the term for the self-activity of that which senses or perceives or imagines, etc. No peculiar or distinct mental property is thus involved.

The error of thought is patent enough in a more concrete instance of it. A dog for example is made up of muscles, glands, nerves, blood vessels, skin, bones, etc. It would be possible to take each of these various constituents in turn and having thoroughly examined them to claim that we have satisfactorily disposed of the dog. Consequently there is no further need to give any significance to the dog as such. But surely it is reasonable to claim that when the animal is pursuing a rat it is not just a conglomeration of nerves, muscles, skin, bones, etc., that is moving in the direction of another smaller conglomeration of somewhat similar constituents, but that the movements are being executed by the dog. It is the dog and not his bones or skin, nerves, etc., that is pursuing and it is a rat that is trying to escape. Moreover the dog is not an addition to his skin and bones, etc. He adds nothing to the size or volume of his constituents. Analogously in claiming separate consideration for volition in the case of human behaviour what is being claimed is not the existence of a faculty or function additional to sensation, perception, etc., but the recognition of the self activity of that which senses or perceives.

We are exposing here once more the persistently recurring fallacy of hypostatization. For there is no such thing as a sensation or a perception or a memory in itself. We may search the brain with the most delicate instruments and fail to find them. For a simple reason. They have no separate or tangible existence. Sensation, perception, memory, imagination, reasoning, etc., are only so many modes or ways of mental activity. And for that mental activity itself volition in its various degrees is a name. It is the self active. It expresses the difference between life and non-life.

On the other hand it is pertinent and instructive to compare and contrast Volition in its highest degree with impulse, volition in its lower degree, or to put it more accurately, volitional and impulsive activity. Both are the self initiative, but with this cardinal distinction. In the case of impulse the activity is of the self but controlled *by* the self only in the lowest degree. For the impulse is given, it is innate or at least not at the moment created by the self, it is already at the moment there, and the activity is prompted by it. Impulse is volition at its minimum. But some measure of it is already there : impulse is not quite mechanical ; it is at any rate *self* activity. The movement is not the result of mere mechanical propulsion. Volition on the other hand, the degree of self activity to which we usually ascribe the term, is activity not only of the self but also by the self, in that it is not the resultant of any urge innate or acquired but is created[2] at the moment. It is free, as impulsive activity is fettered. Because of this difference we may claim Volition as unique in comparison with impulse. But in another sense it is not unique ; for it is out of impulse itself that it has slowly developed. There need have been no discontinuity, for the one is only the other transformed by continuous emergence of one of its aspects and continuous sinking of the other   The determined has been slowly yielding to the determiner.

Meantime impulse continues to survive and thrive. But alongside Volition. Or to put it more precisely volition in human behaviour is now to be found in all degrees of purity. For man ' comprehends ' all the levels that have preceded him. He exemplifies in his own person all stages of activity from the most mechanical, the most impulsive, to the most truly Volitional ; and thus in any actual moment he may be exhibiting volition in different stages of itself.

We have now considered the charge that the introduction of the term volition involves the gratuitous addition of something unique, in the various senses in which the term might apply. In the sense of peculiar to man we have found that man only is capable of volition in its highest degrees of purity, but that no discontinuity need be implied in tracing the rise of Volition from the lowliest animal levels. No sudden interposition of a faculty or special power need be entailed. While if by unique is meant that the concept implies some process or function added to the recognized list of mental modes of functioning, the answer is that so far from adding a function alongside a number of others, we are affirming the existence of something that functions and claiming that it actually does so. We are making the functionings possible. Here is self activity. Of course this self activity may be fairly called unique, in the sense that it is *sui generis* and not further explicable.[3] It cannot be resolved into any other terms than itself. It is as much a mystery as matter is. But of two inexplicables, the electron-proton or energy or matter on the one hand and the self active on the other, why, we may well ask, is to be considered a better or more satisfactory explanation to render the living organism in terms of one inexplicable than in terms of the other ? Why is one procedure supposed to get rid of mysteries and not the other ? Why not explain in terms of both ? In other words, why refuse to recognize volition as well as mechanism ?

(2) *Is the Recognition of Will as an Explanatory Principle a Case of Hypostatization ?*

Since the same argument may be and indeed has been brought against the elevation of intelligence to a position of dominance in behaviour we may consider the double charge together.

That this accusation is unmerited becomes clear as soon as we realize wherein the fallacy of hypostatization lies. The objection to the utilization of abstractions in the explanation of particular phenomena does not reside in the use of abstractions as such ; for after all that is the only means by which the human intellect can explain anything at all. The term explanation is used for the disclosing between transient phenomena of permanent relations which obtain between them, and it is necessary to abstract in order to explain. We analyse the phenomenal appearance and abstract some significant feature of it. We proceed to consider the abstraction. If all that is meant by hypostatization is the using of abstractions in the process of explanation, then hypostatization so far from being a fallacy is an indispensable instrument of all thinking. And all thinking would be *per se* fallacious.

The fallacy then does not reside in hypostatization as such ; or to put it another way, we have to mean by hypostatization something more than abstraction in order to condemn it as a fallacy. The something more is this : An abstraction becomes fallacious when we take over into the abstracted element something more than we have abstracted, and do not acknowledge the debt. The objection for example to Herbart's ' ideas ' as explanations of the course of mental life is not that he deals in ideas but that in order to make them explanatory he has had to endow them with intelligence and volition of their own—he has taken over with his ideas the rest of the organism. Similarly with Shand's sentiments and Thorndike's neurones. The sentiments as organized systems of emotions become fallacious only when we find the emotions *sorting and arranging them-selves*, as if there were or ever could be emotions apart from the self experiencing them, as if indeed they had some kind of independent life of their own, as if indeed, to go further, they could be *explanatory* principles at all. In treating emotions and sentiments as the foundations of character Shand succeeds in belittling the significance of volition and intelligence only by endowing his sentiments with just these attributes, by mistaking them for the individuals experiencing them. And so with the neurones of Professor Thorndike. He succeeds in evading the intelligent and volitional individual as an explanatory principle only by reading intelligence and volition into his neurones ; and emotion as well. They are satisfied and annoyed ; they select ; they are causative of activity. They possess emotion, intelligence, will. A multitude of homuncules.

And it is significant that the very attributes with which the psychologist in each of these cases has found it necessary to clothe his entities are precisely intelligence and volition : he is obliged to inject them here because he has not found room for them anywhere else in his system, and because they remain to be accounted for. Though anxious in the cause of science to get rid of these uncomfortable and inexplicable intruders, it is yet necessary to allow their influence somewhere for the simple reason that life does not *work* without them ; and his explanations of behaviour will not work either. They will be hopelessly unconvincing. The objectionable intruders are accordingly hidden behind the scene, or introduced carefully disguised.

But how are we as psychologists to avoid the fallacy just indicated ? There is one and only one way to avoid it, and that is by rendering it superfluous. We have frankly to give intelligence and volition their due. There will then be no need to endow sentiments or neurones or ' ideas ' with them ; we can treat them on their own merits. But in recognizing them for what they are we are under no temptation to hypostatize them in their turn, for the simple reason that we need not retaliate on the sentimentalists, the neuronists and the idealists, by refusing to recognize ideas and emotions and neurones, and having to find a place for them inside intelligence or will. There is no need therefore to endow intelligence and will with anything besides themselves. Moreover we can and must always remember that by intelligence and by will we do not and need not intend an abstraction at all ; a point we are most careful to insist on in identifying will with self activity, and intelligence with *our* power to apprehend relations, and not with any existence on its own account. To abstract will as vitalists are changed with abstracting it and to set it apart as a special creative force is to run the risk of hypostatization, if we go on to imply that this force or vital principle exists apart from us exerting it and is somehow explanatory of our volitional behaviour, requiring itself no further investigation. There is no need however to turn this logical somersault.

The answer then to the charge that the recognition of the importance of intelligence and will in human behaviour involves the fallacy of hypostatization just as much as does the recognition of the importance of ideas or sentiments or neurones is this, that since the fallacy consists in adding intelligence and volition to these abstractions because intelligence and volition are not allowed for otherwise, as soon as intelligence and volition are recognized on their own merits the occasion of the fallacy vanishes. The admission of intelligence and volition is in fact a deliberate refusal to commit the fallacy of hypostatization. It is a protest against subterfuge.[4]

(3) *The Will as an Arbitrary Intervener in Natural Processes*

That Volition is the opposite of the arbitrary, being insistence upon law, has already been contended, and

N

need not again be demonstrated here. But to those
who are long habituated to a mechanical view of the
universe, as a closed system of inevitable uniformities,
the mere insistence on, and demonstration of, the law-
abidingness of will does not get rid of the uncomfortable
suspicion that we are all the same countenancing, nay
rather asserting, some kind of intervention in the laws
of nature. And a law cannot at one and the same time
be a law and yet subject to interference. A universe
of this kind must be unreliable. Moreover unpredictable.
But since in fact we can and do predict, and our predictions come true, then these interferences do not take
place.

Now one answer to this objection might be that the
science of psychology does not profess to have solved
all its problens. Psychology is science, not philosophy.
Yet it is precisely because it is science that it is its duty
to recognize impartially both uniform and volitional
behaviour, since physical uniformities and volitional
behaviour both are data of experience. The scientific
psychologist has of course no right to propound an
account of human behaviour which " explains away "
one of the orders of experience any more than one which
explains away the other. Part of this reluctance to
deal fairly with both aspects is no doubt due to the
prevailing mechanical bias of the age : we cannot get
away from our increasingly mechanized environment,
and traditions. We have thus acquired a strong
determining tendency to adopt a mechanistic philosophy
where we ought as scientists to be espousing no
philosophy at all.[5] And in this case where sentiment
has been built up we can scarcely hope to yield our
predispositions very quickly to the persuasion of
reason.

The inconsistency between volition and predictability
may however be only apparent. The charge of incom-
patibility rests upon overlooking an ambiguity in the

terms 'intervention,' and 'interference,' the removal of which may diminish the difficulty which the ' scientific' psychologist experiences in admitting the volitional intruder. The employment of the terms interference and intervention really begs the question at issue. For the terms interference and intervention are relevant objections only if they are used to imply that some upsetting or disturbing of natural laws or uniformities is entailed by acts of Volition. But this is surely a misunderstanding of what actually takes place. For what in fact we appear to be doing every hour and indeed every moment of our lives is not interfering with natural uniformities but making use of them. So far from upsetting them or expecting their disturbance we are doing precisely the reverse : we are confidently anticipating their stability. When I get up and approach the door of my room, I avail myself of a certain uniformity in the movements of the door handle and I rely on the handle being still there and on its behaving in the accustomed way. My volitional action has interfered with no uniformity at all. On the contrary it has taken advantage of a large number of uniformities, and has enlisted their co-operation. Precisely how many and which exactly they are, who can tell ? For there is no man living who can give a complete account of all the laws of nature that are operative in even so simple a movement as the opening of a door. Indeed, no one would be more surprised if these uniformities were upset by his opening the door than the scientist himself, for he least of all believes in magic. Should the door on some occasion refuse to respond to his handling of it, or should it suddenly move off its hinges and advance threateningly towards him across the room, so far as he was true to his colours he would refuse to be merely disconcerted but would proceed to investigate the particular law of nature which was expressing itself in this unusual fashion. Thus every volitional act depends for its execution on the stability of universal laws : we cannot hope to execute a proposed act without this very assumption.

But if it is still maintained that the exercise of volition does introduce any contradiction at all, it is a contradiction that is occurring all the time and everywhere. It is the most familiar fact of our ordinary experience, and therefore one which psychology is bound to recognize as a fact.   There is therefore no reason why a student of psychology should feel uncomfortable about the peculiar arbitrariness of volition, or object to it as upsetting the laws of nature, if he experiences no surprise that the door responds in the usual way when he turns the handle, any more than that it awaits his touch before it turns.

We can now see that the terms interference and intervention are misleading because they suggest an unwarranted connotation.   The persistent fallacy of hypostatization is again being committed.   Laws of nature are not susceptible of interference, in the sense that we can alter their mode of happening.   Nor do we undertake to do so.   All we do is to investigate their mode of happening, to discover, that is to say, what these laws are ; after which we take full advantage of them. So far from interfering with them we set ourselves to give them play.   And we rely confidently on their universality.   Our very confidence in prediction implies this confidence in their recurrence and our genuine belief that no Volitions of our own are sufficient to upset them.

The hypostatization consists in endowing these laws of nature with independent self causation—an unwarranted anthropomorphization.   The law is merely a description of how in point of fact a certain number of events are found to happen apart from the human will.   That is to say physical laws are uniformities of movements which are not found to require the initiative of any known living being in order to be what they are.

We are not of course justified in concluding that they

go on of themselves or are so to say self caused, or that there may not be some kind of initiating agent that sustains them. As students of the science of psychology we are not called upon to decide this particular question. We are concerned in facts of observation. And while we observe on the one hand the existence of these extra-human and extra-animate uniformities, we also observe on the other the contingent character of many natural uniformities, their functioning being dependent upon the initiative of some living being. The door handle does not turn until you or I turn it. The automobile does not leap forth from its garage of its own accord. The electric current in my house does not function until I turn on the switch.

The term ' interference ' wrongly assumes that the door and the automobile and the electric current are making these movements of their own accord, and I come in and disturb them. This is the fallacy of hypostatization : a set of movements of a purely contingent nature have been abstracted from the concrete situation and endowed with self activity ; they are regarded as going on of themselves until man interferes with them.

Yet the very ability of the scientist to commit this error is a tacit admission of the existence of will, in the sense of immediate causation. After endowing the law of nature with self activity, the power to go on of its own accord, man's will is then said to imply some interfering with it. But from what source does he abstract this self activity ? From his own experience of himself. Unless he had that experience already he could have known nothing of it ; and he could not have gone on to transfer it in thought to a sphere of phenomena where it does not belong.

The mechanist in fine effects a magic reversal of the universe. He steals life from life and injects it into non-life. But he does not acknowledge the theft. It is the first duty of the scientific psychologist to restore the stolen properties.   Once we have done this and have grown accustomed to seeing things in their right places we become gradually less discomforted about interferences and interventions in natural laws.   For we begin to realize that laws of nature are not inexorable movements that go on eternally of their own will whatever you or I may do to them, but that they are dependent for their particular performances upon what goes on beside them ; and you and I are amongst those outside happenings.[6]   A racing automobile is not endowed with some mysterious capacity to go on racing indefinitely, or with any determination of its own to do so.   It stops when I turn the switch off.   And if I were only big enough and strong enough I could similarly push the moon out of place or throw the sun into another constellation.

It is, we must admit, exceedingly fortunate for the human race that there are so many of these natural uniformities : hard would it be indeed if we were always doing everything for the first time.   Constituted as we are we depend upon these natural laws on all sides for our own personal development, our skills and our achievements, and our own bodily and mental growth. There must be repetition (the law of uniformity) and there must again be innovations, WILL, for any learning or development to take place.   A stone, a river, or a machine does not develop, because it is so remarkably lacking in the latter.   It cannot innovate, it merely repeats.   But life both repeats and innovates.   Law co-operates with will ; will makes use of law.   Will using law is living, as we know it.   Will is the power to make things happen, to take advantage of natural laws. *I can open the door.*   No additional belief is demanded from the student of a science of psychology in order to admit the principle of volition.   If he persists in entertaining a contrary belief, it is up to him to prove a case that conflicts with his actual experience.

(4) *Inconsistency in the Use of the Term Volition*

The objection may be raised that at one time the term volition is used for action initiated in accordance with impulse or instinctive tendency, at another it is the opposite of this, namely initiation as against impulse that is made the cardinal feature of volition. Moreover by identifying volition with any self activity, e.g. the self activity of a dog running after a bone, or of a garden pea stretching out a tendril towards a support, we have robbed the word of any distinctive meaning.

The objection however has been met by pointing out that volition is susceptible of gradations of level or ' sheerness.' And volition at one level may be in conflict with volition at another. Phylogenetically considered the humblest form of volition, or the seed from which Volition of the highest level will sometime blossom, is already evident in the activity of say the stentor making movements of escape from an uncongenial stimulus. Its movement is apparently innately determined, or nearly so, yet it is more than the movement of a mere machine. There is some measure of self activity present. The organism is not constituted so as to react uniformly to the same outward stimulus, and frequency of the occasion may even lead to change of behaviour. The dog after its bone represents a higher level, for we see him avoiding obstacles and even planning how best to secure the bone. He will fight off another dog before seizing it, for instance. Here there is still more self activity, still less mere determination by the environment. But the act is on the instinctive level. By the time we come to man there has entered Volition or self activity on the highest level, namely functioning in control of and in opposition to impulse, whether the impulse be born of instinct or of habit. But since man comprehends within himself the lower level activities, the phenomenon is often witnessed of one type of volition opposing and over-riding the other.

There is thus both continuity, genetic continuity, and

conflict, actual momentary conflict ; we may indicate genetic continuity by assigning the same name to all manifestations, but of the different levels or stages we may reserve the name Volition par excellence for its exercise on the highest level specifically. Initiative is the common element all through. But since it is most initiative, that is at its purest and sheerest, when it is least impelled by impulse, volition is most clearly in evidence at what we therefore call its highest or most Volitional level. There we have self activity most itself. If these distinctions be admitted the accusation of inconsistency can arise only by disregarding them.

(5) *The Misuse of the Terms Higher and Lower*

Psychology as such, it will be said, has nothing to do with morality ; it is not its business to evaluate ethically the processes it considers, so that the terms higher and lower with their inevitable moral implications are better avoided. We have as psychologists no right to prejudge or obscure the issues by weighting the argument with moral values. To this contention there are two answers. One is that the terms higher and lower are already so commonly used in discussions on evolution that no moral implications need arise. By higher is intended a level of greater variety and complexity of behaviour. It is at this level that Volition is most in evidence and Volition appears in its purest form. There seems then no reason for refusing to use a convenient term.

But there may be another and special justification for the use of the terms higher and lower. If, as has been contended, the morally higher life is the life according to reason or as is here put the life according to intelligence, and if as has also been contended it is its direction by intelligence (or the individual following the guidance of intelligence) that constitutes the criterion of Volition at its highest, in virtue of which the individual is found opposing his impulses, then we are justified in using the terms higher and lower in the ethical implications also. Hence a double justification for retaining these terms.

Moreover we should have arrived at a psychological basis for the moral life. The moral life can be psychologically described : life forwarding its own evolution, the individual on the way to emerge at a higher level. On this reckoning the whole course of evolution has partaken of a moral and ethical character, though at levels lower than those at which we are accustomed to call behaviour moral. But there has been continuity, and the same root principles have been at work throughout. But not therefore inevitability, or absolute predictability, about the actual course which evolution has followed ; something not included in a mechanical scheme has been present and operative all through. There has always been something more. Something which when a certain stage is reached, we recognize as ethical in character. And since this something more is to be seen at its clearest where it has most evolved, as indeed we should expect, it is not by tracing behaviour down through the animate scales, but by investigating life where it is most life we shall discover the principle which is functioning more obscurely lower down. To attempt to interpret human life by tracing life back to its lowest and earliest stages is just as one-sided as hastily to interpret the behaviour of the lower animals in human terms. Help must be sought equally from both sources.

(6) *Volition Not an Illusion*

It has been claimed in the course of our exposition that volition, the capacity of self activity, must be either a fact or a fiction, a reality or an illusion, and that mechanistic psychology neither admits the fact nor explains the illusion. If the experience is illusory it is the business of the psychologist to find a place for the illusion as an illusion in his scheme of behaviour.

To this an objection may be brought that since even

the mechanistic psychologist recognizes the actuality of the experience of volition he cannot fairly be charged with regarding it as an illusion, and therefore cannot be called upon to find a place for the illusion in his system. All that he does is to offer an explanation different from the one given here ; in fact he does undertake to explain it while the non-mechanist does not.

This argument however is beside the point. It relies on an equivocal use of the term illusion. By illusion was intended not that volition was not *a felt experience*, but that it was not *true*, that it evidences what does not occur. The mechanist regards volition as illusory in the sense that while it is an experience of self activity, that self activity is apparent not real : there is no genuine self activity at all. No real initiative. The activity is assumed to be determined by what has gone before and by nothing else. But our experience is of activity initiated by us at the moment, and not the inevitable result of our own past. It is in this sense that the mechanist claims that volition is illusory, but can find no place for the illusion. He cannot tell us why we have this experience of being able to choose our action if every action of ours is determined for us. Why this elaborate hoax ?

On what ground, we may well go on to ask, does the mechanist refuse to accept the experience of volition at its face value, and yet accept at their face value his sensory perceptions ?   On what grounds does he accept one kind of experience and exclude the other ?   Why is the percept to be considered a valid experience but the experience of volitional activity not valid ?

He cannot consistently maintain that it is due to a scientific distrust of conscious processes, for the simple reason that every act of perception is as much a conscious process as every volition is. Every observation of his comes to him through consciousness and in no other way. There is, however, one significant difference in the deliverances of perception and those of volition. In

the case of perception the actual conscious presentation
is not first hand.   When I state that I see a cat in the
distance my percept of cat is the result of a series of
processes mediating and preceding the final judgment.
There is the object or occasion of the stimulus.   From it
pass etheric vibrations (or processes in the electro-
magnetic field) which impinge on the retina.   At this
point something happens—we know not what—and a
nerve impulse different in nature from the vibrations
passes inwards to the brain.   In the brain again something happens—we know not what—and there occurs a
sensation, again different in kind from the impulse as
the impulse is from the vibrations.   The sensation has
next to be interpreted before the final perception results.
We are reminded of the children's game of Russian
Scandal, in which a player at one end of a row whispers
into his neighbour's ear a message which is similarly
passed on in succession till it reaches the end of the row,
when the difference between the eventual message and
its original gives rise to merriment.   But whereas in
the game the message is throughout the same kind of
message passing through the same kind of media, in that
of the percept the message is rendered in a new code and
passed on by a different kind of medium at two points
along the line.

Contrast with this the experience of volition.   It is
an immediate first hand experience subject to none of
these distorting media.   Why then are the end results
on consciousness of a process of complicated Russian
Scandal considered more scientific and more reliable
than the immediate deliverances of consciousness itself ?
Why are we to trust the first and mistrust the second ?
In both cases we are accepting or rejecting the deliverances of consciousness ; but in the case of volition there
has been no preliminary contrivance which may distort
the message.   Surely the burden of proving the percept
the more acceptable and valid experience falls upon the
mechanistic rather than that of proving the validity of

the volitional experience upon the non-mechanistic psychologist. If the former are not illusory, how much less illusory must be the latter.

It is no answer on the part of the mechanist to expatiate on the difficulties of introspection or on the unreliability of purely subjective and therefore individual experiences. We may admit that the observation of the volitional experience is difficult, since it is not only subjective but lacks that clear-cut definition and stability which marks for example visual percepts. But the difficulty of examining an object is no reason for denying the existence of the object : volition is not invalidated because it is hard to introspect. We do not regard a poem as more illusory than a plain statement of fact : a thing is not the less there because it is difficult to dissect. The question immediately at issue is not whether there are difficulties in the way of pursuing the science of psychology, but whether the immediate conscious experience is valid. If it is, and we have given reasons for preferring it in validity to external observation, then it is the business of psychology to admit its significance in human behaviour.

(7) *Why Prefer the Martyr or the Hero to the Big Business Man as Instances of Volitional Behaviour in its Purest State*

The question may be met by a clear understanding of the true significance of ' principled ' behaviour. A distinction has been drawn between impulsive and intelligent behaviour and the importance of observing it has been stressed. At the same time in actual life there is probably no instance of behaviour that is wholly either one or the other : the distinction is one of degree, just as the distinction between volition is one of degree passing into what we may fairly call one of kind when we contrast the extremes. The reason why the martyr and the hero have been selected as crucial examples of volitional behaviour is that in their case there is the least

of impulse and the most of intelligence in direction.
There may of course be instances of great financiers, and
no doubt there are, whose actions arc determined
primarily by the most comprehensive principles of which
they are capable, with the least admixture of say the
impulse to self assertion or mastery or personal
aggrandisement. But it will surely be admitted that
in big business these instinctive tendencies or dispositions
are constantly being evoked, and that they, with whatever addition of intelligent principle, do constitute part
of the blend of motive of the individual. Just so far
as the individual is moved by instinct he is not moved
by the highest type of volition : he remains the
instinctive ' natural ' man.

The point that I contend for above all others is that
instinct, and habit derived from instinct, are not the
sole sources of human motivation ; and that man as a
cause is by that very fact self-motivating. Volition is
self-motivation. Volition at its highest level is the
creation of motive. On no other basis can we admit
it at all. For once we grant that all human activity
is either instinctively impelled or impelled by habits
derived from instincts, the volitional consciousness
becomes meaningless. It is an illusion, and has no
place in human behaviour at all. Initiation ceases
to be initiation as soon as it is resolved into original
impulse, for our original impulses are given us : they
entail not initiative but its opposite.

Until modern psychology frankly recognizes that man
has attained a level at which he motivates himself apart
from the motivation of innate factors ; and that that
motivation is and can only be intelligent motivation,
we may struggle in vain to prove ourselves other than
determinist psychologists. For we fail to recognize
that man is the creator of his own motives apart from
those he is endowed with at birth. But at the same
time he is not therefore completely unlimited (or
undetermined if you will) in his choice of action. He

can choose between two lines of action, and two only : impulsive on the one side and intelligent on the other. Try if you wish to instance any others. Hence volitional activity in the sense of action according to intelligence is not and cannot be arbitrary or haphazard, for the simple reason that intelligence is the power of disclosing principles which obtain, namely the true uniformities of behaviour. Volition is behaviour observing uniformities in opposition to behaviour as a chaos of conflicting impulses. That at any rate is Volition at its most volitional.

Once the significance of the distinction between the life of impulse and the life of reason is clearly grasped, we understand at once why the martyr is a more typical instance of volitional behaviour than the big financier is. For the martyr represents behaviour according to a principle based not on impulse but on principle as such. He has exercised his intelligence freely, not in the service of impulse.

On the admission of this distinction between the two extreme levels of behaviour, behaviour at its most instinctive and least intelligent and behaviour at its most intelligent and least instinctive, the case for volition versus determinism stands or falls.

Summarily :

(1) There is no *special* sense in which volition is to be considered unique. It is merely a term for the ordinary fact of self-activity, and is thus in degree present in all life. It adds no extraneous factor. No special " vital force " need be posited : to posit this is to duplicate by abstraction, an unnecessary and confusing procedure.

(2) Consequently the recognition of volition and intelligence as factors in human behaviour does not involve the fallacy of hypostatization. Quite the contrary. For the fallacy of hypostatization in psychology lies in endowing abstractions like ideas or neurones with intelligence and volition in order to help

out the explanation of behaviour. The recognition of intelligence and volition is not the fallacy of hypostatization but its antidote.

(3) The recognition of volition, so far from introducing an element of arbitrariness or lawlessness into human behaviour, achieves the reverse. For behaviour is volitional in proportion as it is directed by intelligence, that is by principles which it is the nature of intelligence to disclose. Hence volitional behaviour is behaviour in observance of law.

That volition implies our control of external conditions is of course true. But this control is not an upsetting of mechanical uniformities but rather a taking advantage of them. And this we are doing every moment of our lives. To deny it is to fly in the face of obvious fact.

To take advantage of them does not mean that they cease to operate : in fact it is only because we believe they will continue to function that we take advantage of the belief.

(4) Whether it is the business of psychology to enter the field of ethics or not, the use of the terms higher and lower for behaviour evolutionarily more and evolutionarily less advanced is a convenience justified by current usage and need give rise to no ambiguity. At the same time there may be also an ethical justification for the usage.

(5) The experience of volition is an experience of you or me self-active, that is initiating behaviour. If that experience does not correspond with fact or reality, that is if we only seem to ourselves to be self-active and are not really so, we may speak of the experience as an illusion.

Psychology has therefore to find a place either for the fact or the illusion. Mechanistic psychology fails to do either. The claim that it recognizes the reality of volition because it admits the experience as an experience, and not as an illusion, is no answer ; for the question at issue is not whether we experience the experience or not, but whether it is or is not a 'true' experience, that is are we or are we not really self-active. The mechanist says we are not, but cannot explain this illusion in this sense.

(6) On the other hand he is willing to accept the validity of the data obtained through his sense organs, in spite of the fact that these data are themselves merely effects on consciousness and many stages removed from the objects which first gave rise to them. Volition on the other hand is an immediate and not a sense experience. No reason is given why the mediate and indirect experiences are considered more valid, more indicative of the facts, than immediate and direct experience, nor why consciousness is supposed to inform us 'right' in the less immediate and 'wrong' in the immediate case. In both cases he relies upon the deliverances of his own consciousness. The fallacy appears to be that of misplaced objectivity.

(7) Though psychology as such has no dealing with ethical values, yet so far as it discusses the evolution of intelligence and volition it cannot fail to recognize that the continuous development of the two in harmony is what in the sphere of ethics would be called moral development also. In other words evolution is an ethical and not only a 'natural' process. It is not inevitable nor completely determined. This is the significance of the admission of volition as gradually evolving through the scales of life. To reject this and to explain human behaviour (and indeed all animate behaviour) in terms of instinct and of intelligence serving instinct is incompatible with any but a deterministic view of the universe including life. The issue therefore between determinism and non-determinism depends upon the recognition or non-recognition of the validity of volition in the sense given above.

(8) Reasons have been given why we are obliged to admit it, if we admit any deliverances of consciousness at all. "*I will, therefore I am.*"

CHAPTER XIII

REPRESENTATIVE MODERN TREATMENTS OF VOLITION

THE view of Volition which has been advocated in this essay will be further clarified and we hope made more convincing if we examine in the light of it some modern psychological treatments of the subject ; and in the belief that more may be gained from an intensive study of one or two typical discussions than by a general survey, and by consideration of the evidence of recent experiment, to these we will now address ourselves.

This chapter then concerns itself with an examination of the arguments of Wundt and James in their capacity of psychologists* and of the more recent experiments in volitional behaviour.

I. Wundt's Psychology of Volition

Amongst the motives which influenced Wundt's treatment of volition were the desires to disprove the claims of a faculty and an over-introspectionist psychology and to provide the will with a scientific and evolutionary basis. He is aware as a psychologist of the phenomenal consciousness of freedom of choice in the individual human being, and his task is that of reconciling the existence of this phenomenon with the claims of science.

His disclaimer of the pretensions of a faculty psychology offers us a convenient starting point, since it illustrates what from our standpoint appear to be both the essential merits and the essential defects of his own position. " It is in the doctrine of feeling

---

*As distinct from the standpoint of philosophy.

O

and will more than anywhere else," he writes, " that psychology still wears the pattern of the old faculty theory. And so it has usually taken a radically false view of these intimately connected processes, regarding each constituent as an independently existing whole, which might incidentally, but need not necessarily, exert an influence upon the constituents of the other. Thus first of all feeling was considered apart from its connection with will, and then desire was treated as a separate process, sometimes found in connection with feeling. Further impulse was opposed to desire proper as an obscure desire, in which the subject is not conscious of the desired object ; or, perhaps, as a lower desire, referring exclusively to the need of sense. (That is why many psychologists hold that impulses exist only among animals). And finally these processes are still further supplemented by the postulation of will as an entirely new and independent faculty, whose function it is to choose between the various objects of desire, or in certain circumstances to act in accordance with purely intellectual motives and in opposition to impulse and desires. According to this theory, that is, will consists in the capacity for free choice. Choice in this sense presupposes the possibility of decision between various objects of desire, and even of decision against the desired object on the grounds of purely rational considerations. It was therefore supposed that desire was a condition which precedes volition and that at least in many cases this latter is only the realization of desire in action.

" We must pronounce this theory a purely imaginary construction from beginning to end." . . . . " Feeling is not independent of volition, as alleged ; impulse is not a process which can be distinguished from will, still less opposed to it ; and desire is not the antecedent of will, but rather a process which only appears in consciousness when some inhibition of voluntary activity prevents the realization of volition proper. Finally to define the will as the capacity of choice is to render any explanation of it impossible from the outset. Such a capacity presupposes volition as its antecedent condition. If we could not will without choice, i.e. as directly determined by internal motives—a volition involving choice would necessarily remain impossible."[1]

Thus Wundt it will be noticed maintains :

(1) That there is no entirely new and independent faculty (independent of our impulses and desires) of choosing between and even in opposition to impulse and desire ;

(2) that in fact the exercise of will in opposition to impulse does not occur ; and

(3) that impulse is not a process which can be distinguished from will.

How far then is the first of these contentions true ?

Is will independent of impulse and desire ?

The question may mean :

(a) Is will or volition a new capacity or faculty possessed by man in addition to, and super-imposed upon, impulse and desire, and not growing out of them ? Is it a separate addition to our mental armoury, a new bit of mental furniture which somehow has fallen to our lot ?

(b) Does it operate or function (do we will) irrespective of, uninfluenced by, our desires—as if, so to put it, they were not there ?

(c) Is it independent of our desires in the sense that we in virtue of our will free ourselves from determination by our desires ? Do we when willing determine ourselves as distinct from and as opposed to the direction of impulse and desire ? Is will, or does will supply, a separate ' motive ' ?

To the first two questions we may join with Wundt in giving the answer ' No ' ; but where we differ from him is in our answer to the third. It does not follow that, because will has evolved or developed out of impulse and represents a later and more advanced evolutionary stage, therefore it is indistinguishable from impulse and never opposed to it. Evolutionarily volition in our view is in the direct line of ascent (not descent) from, and a conspicuous advance upon, impulse ; while at the same time it is only in relation to some felt impulse that volition functions at its highest. The theory that the function of volition is to choose between objects of desire or in certain circumstances to act in accordance with purely intellectual ' motives ' and in opposition to impulses and desires is quite compatible with the view that volition has evolved out of impulse and may co-exist alongside of it.

Wundt's concept and ours are alike in regarding volition as a later development out of impulse, but they differ in this—to Wundt volition is impulse and nothing more, though in its highest form it is impulse manifested under complex conditions ; whereas to us though volition in its lowest evolutionary stage is identical with impulse, yet at its highest level, where it acquires its distinctive name, there have also emerged distinctive characteristics, in virtue of which it may fairly be claimed to be different in kind from impulse, not only in degree or in the circumstances of its manifestation.

To consider the distinctions which Wundt draws between volition at its higher and its lower stages. They appear to be two :

(1) At its lower stage the ' motive ' of the action is simple—impulsive behaviour is an immediate response to an external stimulus or impetus. The action is thus uncomplicated, the motive to it being provided by some external happening. Contrast the complex case when a set of motives present themselves together—the subject is more or less aware of them or at least experiences their conflict till one or other survives and issues in its appropriate action. This is the stage of volition proper.

(2) At its lowest stage the motive of the action is immediate—the individual responds to a motive or stimulus present here and now with a response characteristic

of that stimulus. The event is uniform. But at the highest stage we have no guarantee of such uniformity for the act is determined not only by the stimulus or impetus of the moment, but by "inner dispositions" to this or that type of action which have gradually formed themselves out of previous responses in the past, so that in addition to the primary impetus there is a 'set' of which the subject may not be clearly conscious, toward a typical behaviour pattern which may reinforce the stimulus or may oppose it. In other words volition proper—behaviour in which we appear aware of self-activity, of ourselves determining our line of conduct—is characterized by :

(a) Complexity or conflict of impulses.

(b) The influence upon behaviour of some permanent set or sets.

In distinguishing those stages Wundt writes :

" The facts comprehended under the term will constitute the links in a chain of development. The lower stages of this development, simple voluntary acts, were classed together as manifestations of impulse ; the higher stages, acts of choice, as those of volition proper.

" An impulsive action is one . . . which is universally conditioned ; there is only one motive present in consciousness. Volitional action rises from the choice between different motives, clearly or obscurely conscious." [2]

We may note the manner in which Wundt continues :

" In impulse, therefore, the feeling of our own activity is less developed than in volition ; whilst since the latter involves a decision as between various conflicting motives, the feeling of our own activity rises in it to that of freedom."

We will turn to his explanation of the origin of the feeling of freedom later.

We experience the same cause of misunderstanding as Wundt in using the term volition in two distinguishable senses ; while sustaining this double reference for the same reason, namely that there is no sudden or wide gap at any point along the line at which the mental processes corresponding to the two uses separate and differ. Like Wundt too we distinguish two stages in the evolution of volition, of which the earlier is the stage par excellence of impulse. On the other hand we also agree in designating the later stage that of volition proper, volition in its later (and as we would add, in its higher) manifestation, volition as the ordinary man might think of it ; as for instance where we find ourselves (seemingly at least) choosing between different contemplated actions, and (so it appears to us) really choosing. But at this point we differ. The claim advanced in this essay is that for the psychological scientist the choice should be regarded as a real choice between variant possibilities ; whereas Wundt claims in effect that it is illusory. He has in consequence to explain the feeling of choice—how is it we come to feel ourselves choosing.

His explanation derives from :

(1) The greater complexity of the volitional (the strictly volitional) situation ; and

(2) From a difference in the origins of the motives for action.

As regards the immediate mental situation, the characteristic of the lower volitional stage—the stage of simple impulsive action—is according to Wundt singleness of motive ; and consequently absence of conflict. The individual's action follows the immediate prompting, since no other intervenes ; and therefore there is no need even for the appearance of choice. But at the stage of volition proper the mental processes are more complicated. At a certain stage in his development, the individual becomes capable of entertaining (being aware of, or at least being influenced by) more than a single motive : he may be moved by several impulses at the same time and in different directions. Hence, according to Wundt, arises the consciousness of conflict. And since in the end one impulse wins, we have the phenomenon—the appearance—of choice, for the ' winner ' amongst motives is in a sense ' selected.'

Secondly there is a difference in the source of the deciding motive. In the lower volitional stage, if I understand Wundt correctly, the individual's action is a simple response to some simple immediate situation, and is determined by that situation and the individual's original (unacquired) impulses. So far there is no supplementary influence since experience has left no dispositions to act otherwise. But in volition proper besides the immediate response tendency, there enter dispositions, tendencies to act thus and thus in certain situations, contracted as the outcome of past experiences and determining or disposing the individual to his behaviour even though he be unaware of it. Moreover, this more deep-set disposition may conflict with the immediate tendencies to response. If we then ask further of what are these determining sets the resultant, the answer is that they are sets stamped in the organism through practice by previous acts of impulse ; they are as it were the permanent residues of impulsive conduct in the past.[3] But inasmuch as they arise at the moment from the inner man as he has continuously developed from his past, they bear the resemblance of self-activity, for, after all, they represent, and derive from, a self—a more permanent and more stable, a more ' total ' personality[4]—than would a response determined by the immediate situation and momentary impulses alone. Hence we experience on the one hand the consciousness of choice (because of the conflict and its ' resolution ') and on the other the consciousness of freedom as self-activity (a permanent and more real you and me than the immediate impulsive person being the determiner).

We have now to examine the validity of these contentions. We may put two questions :

(1) Is the presence of conflicting impulses or motives

and the eventual survival of one (or one group) of them a sufficient basis for the occurrence of a consciousness of choice ? Wundt thinks it is.

(2) Is the occurrence of a conflict of impulses a necessary condition for the occurrence of choice at all ? Wundt holds that it is.

To take the first question. To describe the conscious-ness of choice as occasioned by the emergence or survival in consciousness or predominance of one amongst several impulses, and equivalent to our consciousness or aware-ness of that impulse eventually prevailing, is to miss the distinctive characteristic of that state of consciousness. When, torn between fear of death and fear of the contumely of my fellows, I decide in the hour of peril to let the women and children go first ; or when between greed and sympathy (the desire to please myself and the desire to gratify a friend) I set aside my last glass of champagne for his entertainment, or when, in spite of curiosity, I avert my gaze from the telegram left care-lessly open on the table, true as it may be that I feel the urge of impulse, of more impulses often no doubt than one, it is quite untrue to say that my consciousness of choice, when I turn aside my gaze or set aside my glass, is merely my consciousness of one or other impulse becoming stronger. The characteristic quality of the ' choosing ' consciousness is otherwise. It is an immediate awareness of " me choosing," " me deciding," " me placing myself on one or other side." Moreover, I may be and frequently am aware of my choice falling on the side of the weaker impulse. That is one class of case in which my consciousness of " me choosing " is most definite.

Thus the actual consciousness of choosing is not comprehensible within Wundt's terms, which leave its essence unexplained. If the case is one of the ' stronger ' impulse really winning on every occasion, why this consciousness of choosing at all, if in fact there is no *choice* in the matter, any more than a weather cock amidst variable and conflicting breezes can be said to choose whether it will point to east or north or west. What Wundt in effect explains is why there should *not* be such consciousness of choice ; but why there is such consciousness he leaves a mystery.

To turn to the second question : " Is the occurrence of a conflict *of impulses* the necessary condition of the experience of choice ? "

We have seen that when strong impulses impel us and we act immediately in line with them we are likely to be, and usually are, less aware of ourselves choosing our actions than when impulses conflict and we ' choose ' as we say between them. (The process is not really one of choosing *between* impulses, but of choosing between lines of action. But we may pass that for the moment).

But we may now ask the further question whether the occurrence of a conflict between impulses if a frequent is also a universal condition of choice and consciousness of choice ? Is it not also true that we may be just as aware of choosing when there is little or no conflict *between impulses* as when this conflict is marked ?

The answer surely is clear. The universal condition of choice in action is not the co-existence of different impulses but the presentation in consciousness of variant lines of action. We choose when there is more than one object or action to choose from. When my child presents me a box of assorted candies and I pick out the pale pink cream in preference to the chocolate or marzipan I am just as much aware of choosing as when in the interest of my digestion I decline the dainty. But notice how little the sense of conflict corresponds with the consciousness of choosing. In the first case I am all intent on choosing, but the conflict is comparatively slight : I am engaged in selecting from amongst a number of ' pleasures ' all much on a par : but in the second the conflict may be far keener, for I am resisting my impulse of greed, but I am no more aware of choosing (perhaps less aware) than in the first.   Choice was more in evidence, conflict perhaps even less.

As against one class of situation then in which consciousness of choice is likely to be marked—that in which we are torn between different impulses, pointing in different directions—there is also its opposite, the situation in which our impulses are of a kind, pointing in much the same direction, rendering it difficult to choose between objects to all of which we are so nearly equally impelled.   In the one case the choice is difficult because there is conflict, and it is in enforcing the choice upon ourselves that the difficulty occurs ;   in the other the choice is difficult because there is no conflict, and the difficulty lies in making a choice at all.   In both situations awareness that we are choosing, that we are responsible for the choice, is evident ;   it is on the business of effecting a choice that we are intent.   In a word the absence of a conflict between impulses may be as favourable to the presence of choice as the presence of conflict between them :   the impulses may diverge or they may converge.   If this be so then the occurrence of a conflict of impulses is not a necessary or universal condition for the occurrence of choice.

If it were still replied that even in the ' convergent ' case some degree of conflict were present, so that Wundt's contention still holds, the objector would fairly be chargeable with maintaining his position by confusion of meanings ;   namely by confusing an awareness of conflict between impulses with awareness of several different or possible objects of choice or lines of action. Place before me all the letters of the alphabet and tell me to choose one of them.   I at once pick on M, for no reason that I know of, and with no consciousness of conflict.   But I am aware of the existence of twenty-six different possible choices, of which I make one.   Place again before me the alternative of joining in a favourite game or of letting another do so, and besides the aware-ness of alternatives there is consciousness of conflict—an additional and distinguishable mental event. In short though conflict cannot occur without different or alternative actions to choose from, choice may occur without conflict, and (luckily for our peace of mind) often does.

Secondly, it is difficult to acquit Wundt of a much more serious error, that of representing the alternatives before consciousness as of the same general kind. The conflict issuing in volition (of the higher level) is regarded as one between impulses or desires of which we are more or less conscious. But this misses the distinctive fact about volition at the higher level. When I deliberately inhibit the impulse to make a handsome profit by some secret and undiscoverable sharp practice, it is quite true that in making my choice of action I may be influenced by greed on the one hand and fear of social contumely on the other. But it may also have happened that the opponent to greed may not have been the impulse of fear, or that such fear as there was may have been far less impelling than the greed. What may have happened is that in spite of the impulses of greed and fear and in spite of the fear being less than the greed I chose not to cheat ; I preferred to act honestly. And if asked further why I did not seize my opportunity, my answer might have been that it happened to be against my principles. In other words the conflict was a conflict not between one impulse and another (whether natural or acquired) but between impulse and principle—something different from, and often opposed to, impulse. To make his case consistent Wundt would have to maintain that action on impulse and action on principle are psychologically the same in kind, that there is no psychological difference between yielding to the strongest of several conflicting impulses (fear, hunger, anger, etc.), and deciding in spite of impulses to abide by some accepted principle or rule of conduct.

To be clear about the difference is however so important for a right understanding of volition at its highest level that though the topic has been developed elsewhere I make no apology for reverting to it. One difficulty in appreciating the difference—the actual phenomenal difference in quality of consciousness—is that in most concrete cases of choice of action our motives are mixed. Using the term motive for any inner prompter to this or that activity (a mental prompter as distinct from a physical or physiological) the fact is that even in cases in which one believes oneself to be acting on principle, some degree of impulse is usually also operative. In such mixed cases nothing is easier or more likely (the familiar process of preperception) than for the introspecting observer to pick out whichever of these two constituents he is already disposed by habit or training or partiality to look out for, and to claim that *that* element is the decisive factor. Few of us probably realize how readily we commit the fallacy of the single motive. In the world of sense phenomena it is much easier to hold apart the constituents in a concrete whole, for after all we can see the parts of a chair and hear (though with less facility) the notes in a harmony, or taste the flavours which make up a spice. But even in the sense world distinctions are not always easy. Far harder is it to hold and retain apart the elements which constitute a passing psychic state, when the mind is at once observer and observed. The consequence is that in recognizing and attending to one element we are apt to lose hold of the rest, and where in a blend of motives one has been proposed to us, to mistake it for the whole.

It is upon this proneness to over-simplify and upon the difficulty in disentanglement that the mutual misunderstandings of mankind largely depend. The fallacy of the single or partial motive—the tendency to mistake the part for the whole—is a prolific occasion of suspicion and mistrust, and in the concourse of nations a persistent abettor of war. It is the greatest weapon of the religious revivalist, the stump orator, the astute lawyer, the partizan politician and the medical quack. It is also the frequent pitfall of the psychologist in search of truth.

I find my little son, whom I have just forbidden to do it, throwing papers in the fire. Promptly I punish him. I say I do it from a sense of duty—on principle. My wife tells me I gave way to anger ; and I feel some justice in the comment. After all there was some resentment at not securing obedience, at a slight to my authority. In point of fact, however, both principle and ' prejudice ' combined. My action was partly impulsive and partly ' willed.' Further analysis would have shown me impulses also against as well as for my choice of action, for I incline to inertia and I am fond of my son. How often has one looked the other way rather than take notice of some peccadillo. Many impulses no doubt preceded the final action.

But *post hoc* is not always *propter hoc*—in the medley of antecedent and accompaniment the genuine determiner escapes observation. That determiner may be oneself.

For what do we mean by " principle opposing impulse ? " We must beware of giving body to abstractions and of treating them as if they were separate entities or forces somehow operating in human personalities. Strictly speaking there is no such thing as you or I being determined by impulse or by principle in our conduct—we are not one object or event, and impulse or principle another. We must not be misled by language built upon analogies from the concrete physical world. What really happens is that you or I, afraid or angered or feeling tender or inquisitive, act in accordance with our ' total ' emotion ; or again that though afraid or angered or tender or inquisitive, one is also aware of some rule of conduct one has apprehended and accepted and in spite of fear, wrath, love or curiosity, acts on that rule of conduct and not just as emotions prompt. But yet—and this is the point of importance—in both cases it is ultimately you or I that determine or choose the act, you or I that act, and not the impulse or the principle. Ultimately we are our own motivators : we actuate our own choice ; we initiate the act, we determine our own actions. We live.

But between acting as impulsive and acting on principle there is this fundamental difference : when acting on impulse we are acting on a lower level of self-activity—lower as evolutionarily less advanced, waiving the question of ethical quality—we are more determined so to speak and less determining. For in action on impulse the impulse is *given*, it is what we experience not what we create ; while in action on principle we have set up our own ' motive ', we have adopted a guide to behaviour other than the guide that we possess through the accident of circumstance or birth. In action on impulse we allow ourselves to be determined by the given, though we *need* not do so ; in action on principle we originate the determinant ourselves. In neither case are we obliged to act as we acted. But in the former we are more nearly determined than in the latter. In the latter we are more nearly free. And to this difference corresponds a difference in the quality of the conscious state. It is a psychological difference.

Though action on impulse and action on principle differ fundamentally in the determining motive, it does not follow that in a concrete case the acts themselves are different. Impulse and principle may, and, luckily for our peace of mind, often do point in the same direction. The professional worker may like his publicly useful work ; and we mostly enjoy our very necessary meals. Principle and inclination harmonize. In such cases the higher self-activity is less in (conscious) evidence—only when work grows irksome do we force ourselves " on principle " to continue. And even in such a case so intertwined are our motives, that we may be doubtful how much of each is there and how much one factor exceeds the other.

In contrast with our account of volition Wundt contends that we have no power of acting in defiance of impulse, action in defiance of impulse is merely apparent, the fact being that as the individual matures he does not set up principles rationally arrived at but acquires dispositions or sets developed by practice from previously experienced impulses ; and these, though he may be unaware of it, rather than an act of volition or of separate choice, are really the determiners of our conduct when we seem to ourselves to be defying the felt impulse of the moment and to be inhibiting it.

To this we bring the following objections :

(1) Wundt fails to account for our consciousness of exercising choice, which is just as much a psychological phenomenon as anything else, and must therefore find a place in any psychological system.

(2) He fails to account for that feeling or consciousness of a self mastering impulse, of intense self-activity at moments when volition, as we describe it, is most intense.

(3) He provides no psychological basis for the universal human attribution of responsibility, praise and blame, which assumes the agent, and not things that happen to him, to be at the moment determining his own action.

To Wundt's objection that such choice is *ipso facto*, chaotic, arbitrary, inexplicable, the reply is that it is nothing of the kind. For all behaviour is either impulsive or intelligent, or some blend of the two : there is no such thing as merely chaotic behaviour, behaviour attributable psychologically to the individual acting completely at random. We are constitutionally incapable of acting other than as impulse prompts or as intelligence discloses. An act which is not impulsive must be intelligent ; and an intelligent act is one in accordance with some principle, some uniformity, some rule—in a word an act in committing which the agent relies upon the event and upon its being of a particular kind with a particular end result for reasons not dependent upon the agent alone, but holding irrespective of his will in the matter. If I water a plant to make it grow that water is followed by growth is law irrespective of me. I did not ' make ' it ;

but I utilize it for the sake of my garden. Intelligent action is not chaotic but cosmic, it is orderly action initiated by an orderer. There are no acts which happen for no reason and break out anyhow, any when, anywhere. Such action is outside human experience and unimaginable. No one could describe a case if he tried to.

The psychological alternative is one between acts in which we exercise less and more freedom, less and more choice ; a completely free act in the sense of one " all chosen " does not occur.⁻ But acts or events happening to or within us in which we have no choice do occur. My blood goes on circulating or a brick falls on my head, irrespective of any choice of mine at the moment. Here events for us are at the most mechanical. Above that level acts occur on impulse, as when I fling out in anger or flee in fear. But there is choice here, for I need not so have acted ; there is some measure of freedom exercised. Yet in impulsive action we do not exercise our fullest freedom of choice, for we do not choose the motive for our action   We act in accordance with a given motive, an impulse inherited or acquired, at any rate habitual   In intelligent conduct we exercise our fullest freedom ; we choose our reason for action ourselves ; it is not one inherited or habitual as such. We do not act just habitually. We are furthest away from the mechanical level. We exercise the most initiative we are capable of. We do not abide merely by the innate impulses of the race : we do something fresh.

Human responsibility Wundt contrives to explain on his terms by a logical subterfuge. In discussing the causality of will he posits the existence and potency of a " personal factor."   " Personality is the only immediate cause of action."⁴ But when we ask what precisely this means, we are told that very likely we should find at the very beginnings of individual life the nucleus of an independent personality, not determinable from without because prior to all external determination.

To this we may assent, but to establish our freedom of action, our being responsible (in the sense of praiseworthy or blameworthy or held to account) for our own actions, it is not sufficient to refer our acts simply to ourselves, to inner antecedents, if at the same time that self and those antecedents are themselves previously determined by something outside themselves, outside their control. I am not free, because the mechanism that controls my acts happens to be inside me and not without. I am free only if I control that mechanism. In other words self-determination—and responsibility in the sense of accountability for my acts—is simply destroyed if I that determine am determined in my determinations. Having made out a case for responsibility in the sense in which an open gate may be held responsible for a truant cow, or an inherited weakness for rheumatism in later life, we must not then identify it with responsibility in the fuller sense, the only sense in which it involves freedom of choice, responsibility as accountability for our own behaviour. Thus Wundt by a logical confusion of meanings lends an air of plausibility to his argument.

With his over-emphasis of the power of emotion and impulses in human behaviour and his rejection of the faculty of intelligence, to Wundt all volition is ultimately on the impulsive plane and responsibility is reduced to absence of external constraint, with internal factors left none the less constraining.

II. *William James on the Psychology of Volition*

From the standpoint taken up in this book the discussion of ' Volition ' by William James in his *Principles of Psychology* is significant and illuminating. He appears as an honest thinker torn between two loyalties—loyal as a psychologist to science but as a philosopher to truth. As a psychologist James " wants to build a science ; and a science is a system of fixed relations. Wherever there are independent variables

P

there science stops." " So far then ", he goes on, " as our volitions may be independent variables a scientific psychology must ignore the fact, and treat of them only so far as they are fixed functions. In other words, she must deal with the general laws of volition exclusively ; with the impulsive and inhibitory character of ideas ; with the nature of their appeals to attention ; with the conditions under which effort may arise, etc., but not with the precise amounts of effort ; for these, if our wills be free, are impossible to compute. She thus abstracts from free will, without necessarily denying its existence. Practically, however, such abstraction is not distinguished from rejection ; and most actual psychologists have no hesitation in denying that free will exists."[5]

But what does this policy lead to ? It has led James at any rate in expounding the psychology of Volition to ignore the *Psychological* essence of the phenomenon he sets out to expound, and to render not merely a partial but an untruthful account of it, by attributing to the parts he retains in his explanation characteristics which belong only to the parts he leaves out.

In order to maintain loyalty to science he ascribes Volition to mental elements which function as uniformly as processes in physics, yet ' empowers ' them with faculties which destroy this uniformity in order to do justice to the facts.

For the scientist afflicted with philosophical aspirations finds himself on the horns of a dilemma. If as a scientist he assumes the universal reach of law he denies the validity of our experience of Volition ; but if he accepts that familiar experience, which it is his business to ' explain ', then he is denying the universality of law. Many psychologists, as James has pointed out, prefer the scientific horn—they deny the validity, but are unable to explain our actual experience, of will, our awareness of ourselves choosing this action and not that. They dismiss it as illusion. James, too honest and too insightful to waive the problem, strides both horns of the dilemma at once, but in so doing disavows science as an impartial search after truth. To treat as determined what may be self-determining is to prejudge the issue.

To substantiate these comments we may now examine the devices which James as a scientific psychologist employs to embrace Volition under the mechanistic rubric. His procedure is as follows : Transfer initiative from man to his ' ideas ' ; identify ideas with images ; make images dependent on sensations, and sensations in their turn on stimuli without us. Hence stimuli (the environment) determine our ideas and our ideas in turn our acts. Volition becomes a name for a particular kind of consciousness which accompanies mental halting between ideas, a wobbling or a waiting of ideas before action ; or rather a kind of conscious experience accompanying the culmination of that period in action. The class of sensations, be it added, of which the images provoke willed action are sensations of movement.

Let us now fill in this outline. " The only direct outward effects of our will are bodily movements. But these bodily movements have had their source in involuntary movements, reflex or instinctive in nature ; and when a particular movement having once occurred in a random reflex or involuntary way has left an image of itself on the memory, then the movement can be desired again, and deliberately willed. But it is impossible to see how it could be willed before."[6] In other words, willed acts are repetitions of past involuntary acts. There is nothing new about them. To the question which naturally presents itself how on such principles do we ever *develop* at all, ever come to perform new actions, acquire new habits, or in any way *initiate*, is vouchsafed no answer. Man appears as the non-initiating animal.

The machinery for willed action is provided by images, left in the memory, of movements made previously reflexly or instinctively, movements that are determined for us and not on our initiative. These images or ideas (the words are used interchangeably) result from the sensations originally accompanying the non-voluntary movements; they are " the sensorial consequences of a movement," and are the prerequisites of our voluntary acts.

Two characteristics of the experience of volition James adds to this account of it. One of these is the ' fiat '.[7] In willing we are immediately aware of ourselves initiating action, determining to do this not that, either to get out of bed when the alarm goes or to enjoy another snooze. And secondly, there is anticipation. We will in the belief that we also can, and that action will follow accordingly. According to James indeed Will as a state of consciousness is one form of desire : if we believe the attainment is not possible we call it wish, if that it is possible we call it will.[8] Though we need not agree with James in this distinction between wish and will, for we often wish something possible but do not will it —(the drunkard wishes he were free of his habit but does not *will* it)—we can at least agree that anticipation is implied in will, in the conviction that we can affect our own future. Otherwise we should have no reason for willing.

But to consider the fiat. To the unsophisticated layman the fiat is nothing more nor less than the immediate experience of himself inaugurating action, and anticipation implies his belief in the power to do so. But to James the determination of the action lies elsewhere. The ' fiat ' is not what it seems. The anticipation is not what it implies. A movement made in the first instance non-voluntarily tends to recur as the result of a mental image of it.[9] But why should the physical movement follow upon the psychological image ? James solves the problem by making the image causative. This is his famous ideo-motor theory : the gratuitous transference to an abstraction from our mental life of a power which belongs to the concrete being as a whole.

He thus destroys the essence of the ' fiat '.   In defiance of the immediate deliverance of consciousness—the final court of appeal for all our beliefs—that " phenomenal essence of the will " is resolved into " the inward feeling of a spring let loose which we have when we act after long deliberation ", when we think of an act for an indefinite length of time without the action taking place, and this " felt release of the spring " is " the additional impulse or fiat upon which the act effectively succeeds ". But who or what, we may fairly ask, lets loose the spring ? and is the fiat adequately described as " an additional *impulse* ? "   Do we feel *impelled* by it in the same way in which we feel impelled, say by anger or by fear ? What, moreover, is the function of *anticipation* ?   What is the use of anticipating what is unalterable by our will ? In the machinery of volitional action both fiat and anticipation appear superfluous.

Furthermore, the ' anticipation ' is attributed to the images.   In volition we are told there are ' anticipatory ' images.[10]   As if indeed when the sufferer anticipated cure from his dose of castor-oil, what really happened was that his mental image of castor-oil or of him drinking it —and not the experiencer of those images—had some prevision of the beneficial result.

This personification of our images not only runs directly counter to the immediately experienced facts— we do not in willing experience our images as issuing fiats and anticipating, but ourselves—but it fails to account in particular for anything new in behaviour. For how can an image of a past experience bring about new behaviour ?   James has constructed a piece of machinery for repeating the past, and nothing more.

Yet it is the experience of change, of initiation, of acting unhabitually, that the psychology of volition has primarily to account for.   To rob volition of its essence is to abandon our quest.

Just as topsy-turvy is the conclusion reached about self-activity.   So far from explaining it or finding any

place for it in his psychological system James regards it
as sign or symbol of the opposite of itself : when this
feeling of me active, me initiating is most in evidence,
as when I am aware of inhibiting impulse of my own
will, the declaration of consciousness is the opposite of
what it purports to be, it is me being determined by
the stronger of two or more desires, or by the more
impulsive of two or more ideas.

To the claim that willed acts are only the inevitable
outcome of anticipatory images, themselves the residua
of sense experiences, we may enter the counter-claims :

(1) That the essence of willed action is not that it is
inevitable but the opposite.

(2) That willed action is not the outcome of images
nor determined by them.

(3) That the ' ideas ' which condition willed action
are not images but radically different.

(4) That images are not of themselves anticipatory.

(5) That even the very images which we entertain
are not merely the inevitable outcome of previous sense
happenings, for volition plays a part even in the histories
of images.

The first and last of these claims can be considered
together. That images depend upon sense percepts and
that some sense experience must have preceded every
image without which it could not have occurred we may
grant ; and that to that extent sense percepts are the
condition of images. Further, at the moment at which
any image comes into the mind or rises above the
threshold of consciousness we at that moment have
no say in its appearance : it just happens to us. But
over images once aroused we can and do exercise a
decisive influence of our own wills both on their
immediate and their remoter future. On their immediate
future in that it is open to us to dwell upon an image,
or the object it refers to, or not. I recall—to take an
instance—some unfortunate social *faux pas.* I can
then take one of two (or more) actions. Firstly, I can

dwell upon that image, or more correctly, continue viewing with my mind's eye that unpleasant episode, with accompanying distressful emotions, or I can turn my thoughts to something else, to some object of interest within mental call or from the objective environment— a joke uttered by last night's guest or a book lying before me on the table. But more than this; the rejection of an image affects the probability of its recurrence In that way our immediate inhibition of an image affects its remoter future.

Then even allowing that willed action is the outcome of images, yet, so far as we control our images, our willed acts are not inevitable.

But we are not bound to admit that willed action is the consequence of imagery. This brings us to our second counter-claim.

The relation of image to act is not that of cause to effect. There is no particular act tied to any particular image : the same image—an image of the same object— may be followed by various, and not the same, behaviours; Of course, in as much as we are constantly imaging, some images always occur before willed action ; but :

(1) The act which follows is not necessarily nor ordinarily the correspondent of the images.

(2) An act may be quite different from any image just preceding it.

(3) The mental event to which willed action is most closely related is not an image but *thinking*, which is different and distinguishable from imagery. (Not all ' ideas ' are images).

In the first place, then, images that precede an overt act may determine neither its occurrence nor its character. Of some classes of imagery this is clearly true. To what action am I impelled by, say, my image of the rising moon, or of a butterfly sucking from a flower, or even of a house on fire or a cow eating my neighbour's cabbages ? Not one of these images, I think we will admit, incites to any uniform action *specific* to it. Certainly they do not incite us to an act corresponding to, in the sense of duplicating or imitating, the event or scene of which they are images. We do not feel impelled to rise like the moon, to moo or chew like the cow, to cringe like the cabbage, hover like the butterfly, or blaze like the fire. One is more likely to desire to catch the butterfly or to shoo away the cow or to thank heaven that it is not one's own house that is on fire or to content oneself with reflecting that it does not matter much anyway seeing that one's house is sufficiently insured.

The images, however, of which James stresses the motive force are kinesthetic images—images of sensations of muscular or bodily movement. But if auditory or visual or olfactory images do not impel us to attempt to recover past experiences, why should kinesthetic images be an exception ? Waiving, however, the logic of the matter, let us again appeal to ordinary experience. I have an image—to take an example—of myself running away from a run-a-way horse instead of trying to stop him. But the result of the image is that instead of repeating the imaged experience I feel impelled in thinking of the incident to stand my ground—I feel strongly impelled not to run away on the next occasion, though I may have a sneaking hope that the occasion will not arise. Or again, yesterday I had mince pie for dinner. The pleasing image of myself eating mince pie rises to my mind, but I do not find myself in any way impelled to eat a second mince pie to-day. Enough is as good as a feast, I say : to-day let it be apple sauce. No doubt there are occasions when one does re-enact or desire to re-enact the imaged experience ; as when recalling a past success one tells again (with a different audience) the funny story, or imaging the pleasurable bath (in hot weather after exercise) proceeds to the bath room, or yearns to revisit past scenes of delight or to fight one's battles over again. But when rule and exception are equally familiar to us, how know which is which ?

James admits that his doctrine is not self-evident, that we have many ideas that do not in actual fact issue in action. But the reason for this is not that they are not impelling, but that other ideas or images block the way. In short, the perpetual conflict between images blurs their separate impulsiveness. " Every representation of a movement awakens in some degree the actual movement which is its object ; and awakens it in maximum degree whenever it is not kept from doing so by an antagonistic representation present simultaneously to the mind."[11]

Let us dwell a moment on an ambiguity. By a " representation present simultaneously to the mind " may be meant an image of which one is *clearly conscious*. In this case one can certainly reply that we frequently find ourselves not acting out some imaged movement though also unaware of any counter-image at all, as when I image myself drinking castor-oil, have no counter-image of myself not doing so, and yet feel no desire to drink castor-oil. But if by " present to the mind " is also meant that images are operative though one is not aware of having them, one may well ask what is an image when one does not entertain it and how the hypothesis assuming this possible can be verified ? This intervention of antagonistic representations seems then either disproved by actual experience or an arbitrary assumption incapable of proof. Moreover gratuitous, since the facts can be otherwise explained from common experience. Let us return for example to our castor-oil.

Why is it that I feel no impulsion to take the castor-oil after imaging myself in the act of drinking it ? Surely the answer is that I happen not to like castor-oil. It is not in virtue of an image but of my emotional attitude towards the object, that I act as I act. A certain emotion, or blend of emotions, arises when I image myself drinking castor-oil, and I don't drink it. The emotions, we should also note, are associated not with the image but with something to which the image refers

—the drinking of castor-oil.   The image qua image has no impulsive force.   To impel is not its function.

The psychological service of imagery is not to impel action, but to facilitate thinking ; and this it does by presenting the object thought about in a more readily observable form than without the image, though less observable than with the object itself present.   It helps us think about the object in the absence of the object.   It is the nearest we can get to the presence of the object, when the object is not there:

Willed action, then, though subsequent to mental imagery is neither the consequent, nor the correspondent, of any particular image ; but an image may help us think about some actions we are going to will.

This brings us to the question : What is it that characterizes willed action if we leave images out ? The answer can be given in two words :

(1) Intelligence
(2) Volition.

In his account of willed action James ignores the first and explains away the second.   His account confuses thinking—the exercise of intelligence—with the play of images which beset it ; as do psychologists generally who decry " imageless thought. "

We must revert briefly to this controversial subject. In one sense certainly thought is not imageless—images accompany, and precede, and follow, all our thinking. Though individuals vary in the strength and intensity of imagery and some even seem unable to image in certain sense fields, there is no experimental proof that any thinking person dispenses with images.

It has already been claimed that thinking is largely assisted by imaging ; but this does not mean that thinking consists in it.   In this controversy about imageless thought, as to whether when you have taken away the images from the event called thinking there is anything left, experiments have been invoked to prove either case.   But we will appeal from the experts to the common sense of the plain man confronting again his dose of castor-oil. For it may be that the electric glare of the laboratory sometimes affects the vision. A, the subject in question, prescribed castor-oil by his physician, and having never previously tasted it pours out a dose, puts the spoon to his lips, but on the first contact of it with his palate immediately spits it out in disgust. But on a subsequent occasion he *screws his courage to the drinking point* and swallows his medicine. How did he come to do so ? His own account of the matter seems simple and intelligible enough. He says he was ashamed of funking the medicine and knowing that the dose would do him good made up his mind and took it, although he added, " I do not think I have ever tasted anything so disgusting ! " But in this account of it as given by unsophisticated A there are two elements ignored in James' account of volition. In the first place there is intelligence at work, thinking which is not just imagery ; and in the second, there is initiative or will.

A, it will be observed, had a reason for taking the castor-oil, and a very good reason : he believed it would do him good. But just what psychological process does this belief imply ? Can it be covered by the mere occurrence of previous images ? So far as the castor-oil was concerned, A's previous encounter with it was confined to *not swallowing* it, and his kinesthetic sensations were those which accompany *spewing of the nauseous stuff from his mouth*. And we may safely presume that this image of his previous encounter occurred to him. But the representation of the previous movements did not result in his re-enacting the movement or the scene. Why not ? In the first place because *intelligence intervened*. A was able to apprehend the relation—a " causal relation " we may call it—between his taking the dose and certain favourable happenings in his body. For that reason he resolved to take the oil. Now the point to note here is that no number of images of previous subjective or objective happenings can of themselves constitute the apprehension of relations between objects of thought. Yet without the apprehension of that particular relation A would not have taken the castor-oil.

For an image is an image and nothing more. I may have a hundred images about my mind—I may image a hundred different episodes in five minutes, but mostly without apprehending relations. But when I do apprehend this or that relation, as a result of this apprehension I may proceed to act. Images like percepts foist themselves upon us from every side. Consider the case of percept. At this moment I am perceiving the face of my clock, the different parts of my typewriter, sounds from outside—a bird calling, a train whistling, a boy shouting at play, the flavour of that last cigarette, and the feeling of the pressure of my boot on a hurt toe, and all sorts of things besides. But I am not relating these perceived objects ; perceptions come and go, and I pay them little heed. But now and then I effect a relation, as between the time indicated by my clock and my next engagement ; or between a voice outside in the garden and a child I am fond of. And on those apprehensions I determine my action. They provide me bits of knowledge or beliefs on which I act. As with percepts so with images. A may have had all sorts of images during the castor-oil episode. The handkerchief left in his bedroom, the voice of his physician, the smell of lavender in a friend's garden, the wasp-sting he suffered yesterday, he may have imaged these and other previous sense experiences when considering his dose of medicine. But most of them were irrelevant to his immediate interest and developed no relations. In the case of some, however, that were relevant to the interest of the moment he found himself effecting relations, not indeed between the images themselves, but between the objects of thought for which the images stood. It occurred to him, for instance, that drinking castor-oil brings about an end of stomach trouble In other words, he determined his action, not because of the images but as a result of :

(1) His effecting a relation.

(2) Between objects or events for which images stood.

The thought " Castor-oil cures stomach-ache " is not first an image of castor-oil or of me drinking it followed by an image of that same person without the stomach-ache ; it is not even having the two images together ; it is the mental relating of castor-oil to stomach-ache in a very particular way ; the thinking of stomach-ache dismissal as contingent upon castor-oil. This relating power we maintain is intelligence ; and all initiative as willed action has some act of intelligence ' directing ' it.

But we may exercise intelligence without willed overt action. A may have been perfectly aware of the relation between the oil and the ill, but may have preferred the ill. The new apprehension may not have issued in the new act. Why ? We all know the answer. The will was lacking. Instead of determining his action in accordance with his apprehension, A let his behaviour follow the line of impulse, an impulse of disgust, directing him away from the castor-oil.

But why is the psychologist so reluctant to accept an explanation so patent to the man in the street ? Because it is not acceptable to 'science.' Let us recall James' statement of the position : " A psychologist cannot be expected to be thus impartial," he declares, " having a motive in favour of determinism. He wants to build a science ; and a science is a system of fixed relations."[12]

There is honesty in confessing oneself dishonest. For in effect, James has claimed that science is not an impartial search after truth.

These premises justify the exhibition of fixed relations ; what they do not justify is treating as fixed those which are not fixed. The trouble begins when the scientific enthusiast so trims and tortures the facts to fit his mechanical framework as to produce a distorted structure of the whole. If it is the duty of science to expose the determinate conditions of volition it is not thereby its right to claim volition as determinate. James overstepped his mark. He stretched the part to cover the whole. For intelligence is more than images, and volition than the play of impulsive ideas or impulses.

A word may be added on the role assigned by James to attention in the volitional process.[18] Although he has reduced volition to the level of impulse, being a quality of consciousness which accompanies the termination of a conflict between impulses, he also asserts that the characteristic of volition is an effort of attention. " The exercise of will consists in an effort of attention towards a certain idea. This strain of the attention is the fundamental act of will." But we may not conclude that James as psychologist admits initiative on the part of self as such ; for if we ask what brings about the effort the only answer forthcoming is that the idea occasions it. Ideas impel action. Further, the idea occasions attention to itself. " The terminus of the psychological process in volition, the point to which the will is directly applied, is always an idea."[14] We thus reach an argument in a circle. The essence of will is the effort of attention. The effort is inspired by an idea, but is also directed to the same idea. Will, then, is in essence an idea directing attention to itself or an idea pushing itself into prominence, for what else does this amount to ?

In order to save man from self-determination James has transferred the determination to man's ideas. There is here no self-determination, for these ideas in turn are determined by past experiences which one has received through one's sense organs and which have left behind them corresponding images. These images are the efficient ideas.

Hence, if on the one hand, the only propulsion of the will is controlled by images, so too, is the only inhibition. " The only resistance which our will can possibly experience is the resistance which such an idea offers to being attended to at all."[14] Attention, then, and inattention, are equally functions of ideas, which thus completely control our ' voluntary ' behaviour. Willing whatever it may directly appear to us is just ideas for which we are not accountable, compelling to or from this or that movement.

Thus, even ' voluntary ' attention is no token of initiative, but a function of or resultant of ideas in virtue of the impulsiveness of consciousness. Thus again James, the scientist, saves the situation for determinism. Attention with accompanying effort is an attribute of the process of ideas working themselves into action.

The criticism ventured in this chapter of the line followed by James as a scientific psychologist does not extend to his attitude and his convictions as a philosopher and a moralist. Temperament, moral earnestness, and psychological insight combined to make of James a stout and eloquent advocate of the reality of our choice of action and of the profound practical significance of that responsibility. Moreover in his discussion of the psychology of volition there are parts—for example his famous description of the various types of decision— which clearly lose their point if the choice does not really take place. But when we leave description for argument his scientific conscience betrays him into an exception ; and into ignoring the very essence of the experience under study. For after all our immediate and ever present experience of choice is a distinctive characteristic of human mentality, and a scientific psychology which leaves this out is mock psychology and unscientific (because prejudiced) science. The result was an imaginary *tour de force*—a striking testimony to the efficacy of that very initiative which James was at pains not to recognize.

III. *Experiments with Volitional Acts*

With the claim of psychology to the status of a science it was to be expected that even phenomena so intimate and private as those associated with volitional activity would arrive in time at experimental investigation. Within the last twenty years several investigations have aimed at disclosing what actually goes on " in the mind " of a subject performing an act of choice or volition.

The subject is invited to record retrospectively his own mental processes just after they occur. To the extreme behaviourist—and to any psychologist who would treat psychology as a physical science—retrospective experiments with volition may seem gratuitous and futile : gratuitous to anyone denying volition as a distinctive phenomenon, and futile to anyone discrediting retrospective reports. From the position at which we have arrived that volition (at its highest level) is a ' peculiar ' phenomenon, and that we have no option but to resort to introspections and retrospections in examining it, our criticisms of the experimental approach to volition take a different direction. We find that for the science of psychology experiment is in certain respects of actually less scientific value than the ordinary experiences of daily life, in that the experimental situations are necessarily *less volitional* than common real life experiences, and the experimenter much more prone than the ordinary layman to two kinds of bias, firstly to the bias of some professional ' ism ', and secondly to the inveterate intellectualist tendency to empower abstractions. Moreover, in a science which purports to explain or systematize conscious experience it is that experience unanalyzed that is the final court of appeal : have we or have we not ' accounted for ' it ? For these reasons in spite of the advantages of systematic and trained observation ordinary experience should claim in investigating such a subject as volition even more consideration than the made up situations of the laboratory.

In order to add substance to our criticisms we may characterize briefly recent representative experiments and relate them to our problem.[15] In 1910 N. Ach (of Leipsig and Gottingen) reported an investigation in which his subjects had to memorize nonsense syllables in pairs, and on subsequent presentation of one syllable of a pair to respond not with its fellow but with a rhyme. On the basis of his subjects' reports he distinguished the following constituents of the mental processes involved :

(1) The sensory element—kinæsthetic sensations, feelings of strain, etc.

(2) The intellectual element—representation of the end in view and of means of attaining it.

(3) The essential element—the actual *je veux vraiment*, a felt and lived activity, a consciousness of willing ; an identification of the decision with the self.

(4) The dynamic element or consciousness of effort

This awareness of the self which is active is not inferred but experienced, and is *sui generis* : "Consciousness of the ' I ' is essentially different from any other experience. Moreover, in the moment of energetic will-act a definite change of attitude of the ' I ' is lived."[16] The self is immediately experienced by the subjects at the moment of decision. ' This knowledge contains as an essentially constitutive part the knowledge that the execution of the intended act is the result of the actual moment, i.e. of the ' I really will ' . . . The ' I ' appears as the cause of the action. As a consequence of the knowledge that " I am the cause of this result ", there comes besides, a consciousness of ability—" I have done this by my willing. I am able to execute this task."

In the same year Michotte and Prüm[17] reported an experiment in which the subjects had to choose between adding and subtracting or between multiplying and dividing. The stimulus numbers having been presented they had then to make up their minds which operation to perform, and to describe introspectively the events of this reaction period. Here again the reports clearly indicate an immediate awareness of the self-active, a

Conscience de l'action as the authors name it. To the subjects the presence of this forms a criterion of the voluntary nature of the act. Where consciousness of action is absent they regard the act as automatic not as willed. Other elements in the total state of consciousness—tension, muscular sensations, experience of doubt or certitude, and *les notions*—can be present without the act being considered voluntary.

Boyd Barrett[18] investigating primarily Motivation not Volition as such, incidentally reports introspections of his subjects on the will process. The subjects on this occasion had to choose between liquids with varyingly pleasant and unpleasant tastes. As we might expect where the choice was between two disagreeable drinks the subjects found an effort needed to take the drink. A motive according to the reports may be strengthened by reference to a principle or ideal of conduct : and sometimes this may be an important life-principle, as when the subject thinks " I'd better be consistent " or " Better take the more familiar ". In this way the subject as with Ach and Michotte is aware of himself choosing and himself acting, action on a principle being decided by himself.

There is one experiment of the same type which contests these findings, namely that undertaken by R. H. Wheeler.[19] His subjects had to choose between alternative pictures or phonograph selections. His analysis of the retrospective reports of his six subjects leads him to deny the presence of any unique act of choice or self-activity, these apparent phenomena being resolvable into kinæsthetic and organic sensations, the self-activity and consciousness of self being an interpretation of the actual conscious process and not that immediate process itself. According to Wheeler his predecessors erred through insufficiently penetrating analysis, which if pushed further would have disclosed the assumed consciousness of self as a state of consciousness in which recognition of sensations and images produces a sense of familiarity in the experience.   In Wheeler's view the self—the presumed self—is merely the consciousness of continuity due to recurrence of past effects.   In other words what determines the behaviour of the organism are sensational and imaginal phenomena without initiative of the individual as such.

In a criticism of Wheeler W. M. Calkins[20] points out that his subjects' reports teem with expressions implying reference to the ' I ' as determiner of action ; and that he mixes up the very different processes accompanying self-imposed instructions and instruction imposed from without.   His subjects themselves use such expressions as " I find myself ", " I must ", " I hesitate ", " I was then conscious that I seemed to be in the act of choosing the Barcarolle title ", " I like primitive music ", " Choose the one I prefer ", etc., in their records of their immediate conscious processes ; and they do not analyze these processes into anything else.

Even Wheeler himself recognizes the existence of self-imposed instructions :   " The acceptance of the *Aufgabe* . . . seems to be in essence a motor response either to the stimulus of self-imposed instructions or of instructions imposed from without."   He speaks of the subject accepting self-imposed instructions when in default of others.   A subject " imposed upon himself the subsidiary task to compare two alternatives."

Her contention is that Wheeler has been led by sensationist preconceptions to explain away evidences of self-activity, while accepting as valid the evidence of sensation or imagery.   If both are in evidence both should be equally admitted.

A later investigation by H. M. Wells[21] using, as with Boyd Barrett's experiment conducted under Michotte's guidance, liquids of varyingly agreeable or disagreeable taste, with which the subjects were familiarized beforehand, supports the claim to self-activity as an immediate conscious experience.   The liquids being given nonsense names (to exclude extraneous associations) the subject had then to choose between alternatives and to record just afterwards his conscious processes during the choice. The reports of the six subjects support the view that the ' Self ' is an immediate datum of consciousness. Her subjects were " quite clear and insistent in emphasizing the radically different nature of awareness of kinæsthetic and organic sensations on the one hand and the consciousness of self-activity on the other ". They found it possible to separate the two when

(1) consciousness of ' self-activity ' and kinæsthetic and organic phenomena are present together in conscious ness ;

(2) ' self-activity ' occupies the focus to the relative exclusion of everything else.[22]

So far as the most direct experimental evidence goes it predominantly supports the contention that Volition is not to be regarded as the operation of impulse or a complex of impulses, but as a direct activity of the individual self—the self deciding between objects. If the conflict were one between impulses, with the stronger or stronger combination prevailing, the consciousness of self-activity behind the act of choosing would remain a gratuitous epiphenomenon, supervening upon the play of impulse, an illusory intuition. But there is no more reason for rejecting it as valid material for psychology than there is for rejecting the evidence of sense perception upon which all science relies.

Corroborative as these experiments may be, they are still less convincing than many of our experiences in ordinary life, for they fail to show us Volition at its most volitional. And necessarily. A systematic experiment is a set of performances made to order.

A man executes a choice, exercises his freedom, manifests Volition, most seriously and emphatically when he is faced with what one may call a life situation, when, that is, the alternatives are such as bear importantly upon his permanent interests and welfare ; whereas an experiment contains a situation deliberately separated from life as a whole, and choices that have no special significance for it.   Contrast for example the experiences of a man deciding his life's career, or his marriage, or between riches with honour and poverty with calumny for the sake of a high ideal, with that of A or B or C choosing the more or less disagreeable of two kinds of drink, or resisting a preference for one of a pair of nonsense syllables.   The difference between the two sets of cases is crucial : the degree of self-activity in the ' real life ' situations is out of all proportion to that manifest in the experiments.   In ' real life ' we have an individual (1) for an ideal *set up by himself* resisting (2) of *his own accord* (3) *powerful contrary impulses* towards (4) persistently attractive satisfactions.   In the case of the alternative drinks we have the individual (1) for no important reasons, resisting or not resisting (2) on the instruction of another (3) a comparatively trivial impulse toward (4) a momentary satisfaction.

The experiments also illustrate a second impediment, the proneness, especially in introspective analysis, of the professional psychologist to be influenced by bias.   It is absurd to suppose that Wheeler's six subjects in his experiment should have concurred in experiencing radically different constituents of consciousness from those experienced by Wells' six subjects in an experiment essentially similar.   In experiments on Volition both experimenter and subjects have been for the most part professors or students of psychology, already advanced enough in their study to have espoused some theoretical ' ism '.   And where immediate observation cannot be shared with others 'preperception' or prejudice goes unconvicted.   The professional worker has a pet ' ism ' at stake, and a reputation bound up with it ; the layman, neither.

And thirdly there is the intellectualist fallacy of ' empowering ' the products of abstraction.   All thinking involves abstraction—the attention to and concentration upon elements in a concrete whole.   The fallacy lies not in attention to these elements but in ' empowering ' them, that is endowing with causal efficacy what are only aspects or attributes of a concrete whole. Thus it is that we find among professional psychologists some who treat the external stimulus as initiating our behaviour, some the inner impulse or desire, some images and ideas, or again sensations and percepts, or even consciousness itself. The plain man in his daily practical life escapes this fallacy, ascribes the bulk of conduct to the individual as such—himself or another— and holds him to account for his acts. He rightly trusts his immediate experience of self-activity as authentic, because he has not by thinking split it into separately ' efficacious ' parts.

The fallacy derives from treating the psychical as the physical—To discover what constituent in a chemical compound or mixture primarily occasions this explosion or cures that disease, what in the soil favours the development of this or that plant, we split the concrete whole into its constituent parts and try out the effect of one or other of them. Similarly with the mind : the thinker does in thought what the ' practician ' does in the concrete, and proceeds to ' empower ' the constituent elements accordingly. He thus begs the question at issue, by assimilating the psychical to the physical at the outset.   But our immediate experience—the only final court of appeal—protests and that is why the layman may be right and even the philosopher wrong.

For these reasons we may regard the results of experiments with volitional activity as suspect unless they also tally with the immediate deliverances of the unsophisticated volitional consciousness. What you and I immediately experience is at once the proper material for psychology and its final referee.*

*It is even possible by an effort of abstraction to regard self-activity itself or the whole itself as in some way a determinant of action separated from actual individual people.   One may claim for instance that the experienced self-activity or the consciousness of self-activity effects action separately from you or me—it is our self-activity that does it, not us.   The now fashionable ' Gestalt ' psychology easily lends itself to an apotheosis of the whole or the ' gestalt ' as something in personality that takes charge of our conduct and can be held to account for it.

CHAPTER XIV

CONCLUSION AND SUMMARY

WE may now attempt to draw together the threads of our argument. Our treatment has been concerned mainly with intelligence and volition, because it has been necessary to bring into prominence these neglected and misunderstood but cardinal factors in human behaviour. We have attempted to interpret intelligence and to instal it in its rightful and authoritative place ; and to restate and reinstate volition ; and we have claimed that no explanation of human nature and behaviour that is scientific (consistent in itself and with the data) is possible without them.

It has been necessary also to revert to the debated subject of instinct because human behaviour is largely an inter-play between instinct, intelligence and volition, and we cannot understand the role of intelligence and volition unless we have first considered that of instinct also.

There is however a fourth factor to which we have merely referred incidentally, namely habit. There has been no reason for a special treatment of it, since habit and the mechanistic element in human behaviour generally (for habit is a mechanistic element), is already fully recognized in current psychology, and our interest has been in exhibiting the neglected factors. But inasmuch as mechanism (of which habit is a typical expression) has its share in human behaviour no less than the non-mechanical factors, it will make for completeness if we attempt a description, however brief, of the inter-play of these four factors with one another, for to draw a map of the course of human conduct we need them all.

As regards their relative contribution to behaviour and development these four factors fall into two sets of contrasting pairs. We may pair instinct against intelligence and habit against volition ; or again habit against intelligence and instinct against volition. To touch on each of these contrasts :

A. *Instinct and Intelligence.*

Instinctive impulse unless directly satisfied, prompts the exercise of intelligence, so that intelligence is constantly serving instinctive ends. Hence in any activity the two are inextricably mixed, and we may either reserve the term instinct for that part of the activity which is innately determined or we may claim intelligence as a constant element in instinctive activity. But intelligence also is capable of formulating new ends, in the shape of principles not in line with instinct.

Instinctive ends are stable : it is possible (though difficult) to classify and survey them : intelligent ends are unstable, as intelligence itself turns on its own ends and reveals new ones. Intelligence is a progressive, not a stabilizing, factor, and therefore can propose no final ends ; else it would cease to progress. It formulates its provisional ends through its power (for it *is* that power) of constantly disclosing ever wider and more comprehensive relations, consistence with which in practice is progress in human conduct. In this way, for instance, we pass from narrow egoistic to family, and from family to community, from community to national, and finally to world relations and harmonies as our goals. Thus intelligence supersedes impulse as our guide : there are family instincts, but no instinct to international harmony. To supersede instinct is not of course always to suppress it.

B. *Habit and Volition.*

Habit is the expression of the mechanical tendency in human behaviour, the tendency to sameness or repetition. It is itself the resultant of repetition, being the strengthening tendency to go on repeating. It serves to stereotype or fix behaviour, and it always reverts to the past, to the old, and so can never ' explain ' or introduce the new. The introduction of the new in behaviour awaits volition, the self-initiating. Volition, not habit, ' explains ' innovation, and is the condition in conduct of all progress.

But habit has here its place also ; for acts of volition begin to pass into habits directly they occur—there enters at once the mechanical tendency, namely, to repeat. Moreover volition without habit would be futile, it would move nowhere ; while habit without volition would not move at all. Progress, development, learning, depends upon a nice adjustment or equilibrium between the two. Volition inaugurates, habit consolidates, advance. The individual of routine, the old fogey, the mere conservative, is over habitual ; the random enthusiast, the reckless genius, the mere radical, is over volitional. All sure development of individual or community depends upon maintaining rhythm between the two.

C. *Habit and Intelligence.*

As volition is the self initiating in conduct, so intelligence is the self initiating in consciousness. On this plane habit shows itself as the reproductive tendency, the same presented ' situation ' tending to ' reinstate ' its former context. Stimulus-response on the ideational plane, the mechanical aspect of mind. Habit therefore can ' explain ' no new ' thought,' just as it can explain no new action. And intelligence does for thought what volition does for action : it introduces the new. It is the innovator, as memory (the reproductive tendency) is the conservator, and the consolidator, of each ' intelligent ' advance. The parallel is more than a parallel, for in the last analysis the two, intelligence and volition, are fundamentally the same : they are life asserting itself as against non-life, life pushing ahead. Both are the self-initiative.

And just as practical habit and volition in alliance make for progress, so is it with memory and intelligence. The mere apprehension of new relations would be fruitless unless we also remembered. But memory, the act of reproduction, would mean stagnation without intelligence. All intellectual progress depends upon a nice adjustment or equilibrium between the two. Fresh thoughts do not fructify if they are quite forgotten. But life is lifeless without the new. Yet it is easier to be too habitual, too reproductive, than to be too 'intelligent' and 'original' : that is where volition has to reinforce intelligence, or where intelligence exhibits its volitional aspect.

D. *Instinct and Volition*

Here again we have both unity and division. Instinctive impulse is the earliest, the most primitive, form of volition. It is self-activity nearer the mechanical level. Yet it *is* self-activity ; for even the paramœcium is not quite mechanical ; its movements are not precisely the same every time. There is some degree of adaptation to varying circumstances. And in plant life the same. No two plants grow just alike. They have some power of self-response. Some precursor of intelligence and therefore of volition already comes in.

Moreover volition, in the stricter use of the term, has emerged out of impulse by slow degrees ; whether by variations or mutations we need not decide. And in man both are motives. The instinctive represents the more mechanical, or at least the more determinate, for instinctive impulses are 'given,' they are so to speak part of the made machinery of the mind. But unlike machinery, these springs of conduct do not have their source without but arise within. They do not merely transmit the original energy of the stimulus. They are thus self-active. But volition is the much more self active. It is the self *wholly active*—not to be confused with the whole self active if we include in the self its habitual and instinctive impulses—the self wholly active, in that it is free from the determination of habitual and instinctive impulses, with which it contrasts and which it may inhibit. It is thus opposed to the given, the mechanical, the determined, the repetitive. Thus out of instinctive impulse has arisen its potential master. If it assert its mastery ; for the power (not the necessity) of mastering impulse is the will.

E. *Instinct, Habit, Intelligence, and Volition*

Man ever following the line of least resistance would be man instinctive becoming man habitual ; for we are forming habits all the time. In such an individual instincts would consolidate as habits. Rendered in terms of instinct and habit, with intelligence and volition left out, the individual would be achieving mechanism. But the share of intelligence and volition in this habit formation saves us from this fate. We can and in varying degrees do take charge of our own habits.

At their most mechanical, habits are seen as simple reflexes, whether ' in-body ' physiological reflexes or reflex reactions to external stimuli. At this level they are below intelligence and beyond the reach of volition. The repetitions go on as it were of themselves. At the level of instinct, though the instinctive impulses prompt, intelligence is intervening or assisting at every turn : habit forms under the joint direction of innate impulse and intelligent volition. Most habits therefore, if not all, express both these factors. It is for that reason that habits are never quite habitual, never quite automatic nor confirmed. We are habitual in more or less degree. The decision is ours. We are making and unmaking, forming and reforming, adding and subtracting habits all the time. The habitual and the volitional are inter-active.

Habit is acquired impulse, just as instinct is given

impulse. Habit is instinct in the individual in the making, yet it may never be made. Nor in the individual is it ever quite established : volition may still resume control. While there is life there is will.

F. *Intellect and Character*

What then is intellect and what character ? Intellect is the triumph of intelligence over the mechanical in consciousness, and character the victory of volition over the mechanical in conduct. Repeated acts of intelligence —repeated discoveries (apprehensions of the new)— result in intellect ; repeated acts of volition (the new in conduct) result in character. But both without mechanical foundations would be the baseless fabric of a passing dream

GENERAL SUMMARY

The main contentions in this essay may be summarized as follows :

(1) Self-activity or initiative as distinct from mechanical movement characterizes life. The movement or action originates in the organism, and is not imparted to it from without.

(2) This initiative has evolved through stages or degrees of which we may notice three, namely, reflex activity (reaction to impact or stimulus, initiative from its minima, comprising various gradations above the mechanical up to the more or less conscious and controlled) ; instinctive or impulsive activity—a stage of response to urge innate or acquired ; and pure self-activity or true initiative.

(3) The first two stages on the way to true initiative distinguish life below the human,* evolving into the third stage which emerges in man, whose behaviour however comprehends all three, and seldom if ever exhibits the third quite pure.

(4) Volition as a distinctive term may be used of the third grade of behaviour, and in its most rigid application

* Bnt the promise of the third stage appears even below man.

when the highest form of initiative finds itself in opposition to a lower : the self controlling or inhibiting impulse.

(5) The capacity of man to originate (initiative) is not confined to overt or motor behaviour ; it also characterizes cognition. In the sphere of action we may call it volition ; in that of cognition intelligence.

(6) As intelligence initiative consists in discovery— the apprehension or disclosure of relations, inter-relations, and systems of relations, not absolute but in reference to ends (' given ', or adopted by the individual). Thus action *qua* intelligent is relevant behaviour in a new situation.

(7) All human behaviour (at least above the reflex stage, unless we include this also as ' impelled ') is either impulsive or intelligent ; usually in any particular instance a blend of both. Man is distinctly lower than the angels.

(8) Behaviour most evolutionarily advanced is behaviour in which intelligence and volition co-operate ; or rather, truly volitional behaviour is action in accord with intelligence (whether impulse be for or against).

(9) This exhibits itself as consistency with or adherence to principle (self-determined, not imposed from without)* and in social life as observance of the golden rule— intelligence universalizing behaviour beyond the Ego (thus passing from egoism to altruism).

(10) Volition, as initiative or self-motivation in action, makes the transition possible.

(11) *a.* Intelligence without volition is impotent ; but volition without intelligence is impossible.

b. The will is free in proportion as intelligence directs volition, i.e. volition in its highest form signifies a free will.

(12) Though volition or initiative in all stages is a familiar fact of daily life, yet this has been obscured by

*Character is an acquired disposition to adhere to principles self-determined in control of impulse.

modern subjection to ' scientific ' or pseudo-scientific psychic dominants, specifically those of mechanism and materialism.

(13) Science taking its cue from its ' successes ' with inorganic nature has mistaken itself for the pursuit of invariable uniformities instead of the pursuit of truth.

(14) In psychology, the science of human activity, where mechanism and initiative, uniformity and novelty, repetition and innovation, impulse and volition blend, this mistake has meant

a. Undue stress upon the first factor in each pair, and upon the evolutionarily less advanced aspects of human life ; and

b. A certain credulity as to the greater ' explicableness ' or finality of some material basic unit of life than of some spiritual or psychic entity ;

c. The entertaining of a number of particular fallacies, e.g. as to the nature of cause, that volition ' upsets ' the laws of nature, that explanation is necessarily mechanistic, etc.—which fallacies gravely hinder the progress of our science.

REFERENCES AND NOTES

CHAPTER I

1 Typical is *Animal Intelligence*, by C. J. Romanes (1883)' cited by E. L. Thorndike in his *Animal Intelligence*, pp. 68 *sqq.*

2 " The historical development of comparative psychology," C. J. Warden, *Psychological Review*, March 1927, pp. 145 *sqq.*

3 *Introduction to Comparative Psychology*, by C. L. Morgan (1894), p. 53 : " In no case may we interpret an action as the outcome of the exercise of a higher psychical faculty if it can be interpreted as the outcome of the exercise of one which stands lower in the physical scale."

The canon seems ambiguous and questionable : e.g.

What is higher and lower in the psychical scale ? Again, supposing an action is the outcome of a higher but can be interpreted as the outcome of a lower, the canon cautions us against entertaining the truth. A dog's barking in its sleep may indicate a dream, but be interpretable as a purely physiological reflex.

4 *Animal Intelligence*, by E. L. Thorndike, first published in 1898 (*Psychological Review Monthly Supplement*, vol 2, No. 4) ; in book-form in 1911.

5 Extreme examples are J. Loeb (*The Mechanistic Conception of Life*) and A. P. Weiss (*The Theoretical Basis of Human Behaviour*) ; but the Behaviourist, J. B. Watson, and other adherents of the Stimulus-Response School, also start out from mechanistic premises. Even professed anti-mechanists are often unduly influenced by mechanist preconceptions. See Chapter IX

6 Symposium on *Instinct and Intelligence*, by C. S. Myers, C. L. Morgan, W. Carr, G. F. Stout, and W. McDougall, *British Journal of Psychology*, October 1910, pp. 209 *sqq.*

7 *Early Conceptions and Tests of Intelligence*, by J. Peterson (1925), pp. 257 *sqq.*

8 " Intelligence and its Measurement," *Journal of Educational Psychology*, Vol. 12 (1921). B. Ruml and S. L. Pressey do not attempt to define intelligence. The latter " is not very much interested in the question ".

9 *Ibidem.*

10 See note 12, Chapter VII, below, for a selection of definitions and descriptions of intelligence.

CHAPTER II

1 *Social Psychology*, by F. H. Allport, pp. 11 and 12. " Consciousness, as we have just intimated, exerts no influence, and therefore explains nothing in the mutual reactions of human beings." Again, " the means by which one person stimulates another is always some outward sign or action : it is never consciousness."

cf. *Psychology from the Standpoint of a Behaviourist* (1924), by J. B. Watson, p. 2 note : " The behaviourist finds no evidence for mental existences or mental processes of any kind."

Also *Introduction to Comparative Psychology*, by J. B. Watson, p. 7 : " The time seems to have come when psychology must discard all reference to consciousness." cf. p. 5 : " One can assume either the presence or absence of consciousness anywhere in the phylogenetic scale without affecting the problem of behaviour by one jot or tittle."

2 *Op. cit.*, Allport, p. 17 : " The energy, or less exactly the object from which it is derived, is known as the stimulus, while the resulting activity is called the ' response '." And p. 147 : " A social stimulus is any movement, gesture, or sound—in short any reaction, made by an animal (human or infra-human)—which produces a response in another."

cf. *Psychology from the Standpoint of a Behaviourist*, by J. B. Watson, p. 10 : " A stimulus is always provided by the environment, external to the body, or by movements of a man's own muscles and the secretions of the glands ; finally that the response always follows relatively immediately upon the presentation or incidence of the stimulus."

3 *Op. cit.*, Allport, Chapter III, on *Fundamental Activities*, pp. 50 *sqq.*

4 *Introduction to Social Psychology*, by L. L. Bernard, pp. 106, 114, 110, 133-9.

" The units of behaviour discovered in this chapter (on behaviour patterns) are random movements, reflexes, instincts and tropisms." " Instincts differ from reflexes in their greater degree of complexity." cf. Watson's definition of an instinct as a " concatenation of reflexes ".

" An instinct is a specific stimulus-response pattern, a neural structure."

5 *Op. cit.*, Bernard, p. 143. cf. Allport's statement of the law of conditioned response : " an originally inadequate stimulus if given at the same time as a biologically adequate stimulus will, after sufficient repetition, suffice of itself to call forth the characteristic response."

6 *Op. cit.*, p. 144. " Ordinarily the simple acquired overt

adaptive readjustment neither originates nor ends primarily in the neural processes. Its inception comes from the presentation of unusual stimuli to the end organs of the nervous system with the result that new adjustments must be formed, at first by the trial and error method."

7 *Op. cit.*, p. 55. " Just why the reflex arcs which produce the successful movements are thus selected and ' fixated ' in this process, while the useless responses do not persist, is not clearly known. A partial explanation may perhaps be found in the facts that the successful response, since it occurs in each trial, is in the end the reaction most frequent in occurrence. It is also the most *recent* (that is, the last used) at the beginning of each trial, because its occurrence marks the termination of the preceding trial. These factors, combined with the reinforcing effects of visceral (emotional) reactions, are no doubt operative in lowering the synaptic resistance and fixating the arcs of the successful movements."

Objections to this partial explanation are :

(*a*) The successful response does not occur in each trial, but may occur only in the successful one, and is repeated after the success not before. That is, the success conditions the repetition not *vice versa.*

(*b*) Since it may not occur in any trial at all, *unless that trial succeeds*, the most recent response after any trial need not be the successful one.

(*c*) No reason is given why visceral reactions should reinforce the effect in the absence of any consciousness of success on the part of the organism (which on Allport's premises has no effect on behaviour).

8 *Op. cit.*, Allport, p. 56. " Thought, therefore, is an abridged and highly efficient form of trial and chance success in the consummation of the prepotent reflexes."

9 *Op. cit.*, Allport, p. 11.

10 *Psychology from the Standpoint of a Behaviourist*, by J. B. Watson, p. 10.

If we exclude consciousness stimulus means only a movement of an object affecting a nerve ending and occasioning an impulse. But psychologists who disclaim the efficiency of consciousness are apt to slip consciousness, against their own principles, into the stimulus, thus achieving plausibility through inconsistency. Both Allport and Bernard for example stress the importance in human behaviour of language. To be consistent they must maintain that whether the words are understood, indeed whether they are even perceived (for perception involves consciousness) or not, makes no difference to our resulting behaviour.

11 *Op. cit.*, p. 62. On p. 64 we read " The outworn pedagogical view that man is a creature controlled essentially by reason divorced from the lower ' appetites ' is rapidly being displaced by this deeper truth. Intelligence is the servant, not the master, of autonomic activities."

12 *Op. cit.*, p. 104.

13 *Op. cit.*, p. 208.

14 *Op. cit.*, p. 209.

15 *Op. cit.*, p. 209.

16 *Op. cit.*, p. 211.

17 *Op. cit.*, p. 212.

18 *Op. cit.*, p. 212.

19 *Industrial Psychology*, by C. S. Myers, p. 52.

" Generally speaking the more intelligent the worker the more irksome becomes the maintenance of the required attitude, because of the demands of his intellectual processes for more varied occupation. An excellent illustration of this is afforded by a recent laboratory experiment where four unemployed work girls were engaged in the daily repetitive work of cross-stitching throughout two months. Of these four girls, two had been rated by an intelligence test as highly intelligent, the third showed average intelligence, and the fourth was distinctly below average in intelligence. Each of the first two girls showed distinct signs of boredom in the work ; the one was restless and yawned, seizing every opportunity for change of posture and engaging far more often than the others in conversation, while the other confessed that she found the work very tedious and would not like to do it regularly. These two most intelligent girls, though capable of reaching a high output from time to time, proved unable to maintain it." Of the other two girls the one third in intelligence did the best work of the four, and neither of them complained of monotony.

CHAPTER III

1 *The Nature of Intelligence*, by L. L. Thurstone.

2 *Op. cit.*, pp. 24 *sqq.*

3 *Op. cit.*, p. 159. " The intelligence of any particular psychological act is a function of the incomplete stage of the act at which it is the subject of trial and error choice. Intelligence considered as a mental trait is the capacity to make impulses focal at their early unfinished stage of formation."

4 *Op. cit.*, pp. 125, 126.

5 *Op. cit.*, Chapter VIII, especially p. 122.

6 *Op. cit.*, p. 157. " Those states of mind in which the

impulse is as yet loosely specified are known as universals. They are the higher thought processes."

7 *Op. cit.*, p. 163.

" Further development of intelligence might give facility in selecting effective behaviour with impulses that are close to their source, while they are in what we know as the preconscious or subconscious. To think would then be to use terms that are less and less cognitive and more and more loaded with affectivity. It might possibly come about that the highest possible form of intelligence is one in which the alternatives are essentially nothing but affective states. Some characteristics of genius would not be inconsistent with such a view."

CHAPTER IV

1 *The Growth of the Mind*, by K. Koffka, pp. 153-74.

2 *Op. cit.*, p. 131.

3 *The Mentality of Apes*, by W. Köhler, p. 180.

4 " Intelligence in man and ape," by H. Wyatt, *Psychological Review*, September, 1926, p. 381. See also " The psychology of form," by E. Rignano, *Psychological Review*, March, 1928.

CHAPTER V

1 This " economy of consciousness " is generally recognized in connection with the establishment of habits ; cf. W. James' *Psychology* (briefer course), p. 139. But the same principle " only that degree of conscious explicitness which serves the purpose " applies equally in the case of first apprehension of relations. For immediate motor reactions (as of the boy sharpening his pencil) the apprehension can be fleeting and almost at once forgotten ; for a reasoned argument or exposition it must be clear and sustained.

2 " The Psychology of Efficiency," by H. A. Ruger, *Psychological Archives*, Vol. 2, No. 15 (June, 1910), pp. 1-88.

3 *Op. cit.*, p. 12.

4 *Op. cit.*, p. 33.

5 *Animal Intelligence*, by E. L. Thorndike, p. 73.

" We may, by a careful examination of the method of formation of these associations as it is shown by the time curves, gain positive evidence that no power of inference was present in the subjects of the experiments. Surely if 1 and 6 (cats 1 and 6) had possessed any power of inference, they would not have failed to get out after having done so several times. Yet they did. If they had once even, much less if they had six or eight times inferred what was to be done, they should have made the inference the seventh or ninth time. And if there were in these animals any power of inference, however rudimentary, however sporadic, however dim, there should have appeared among the multitude some cases where an animal, seeing through the situation, knows the proper act, does it, and from then on does it immediately upon being confronted with the situation. There ought, that is, to be a sudden vertical descent in the time curve."

Köhler's apes it will be remembered, exhibited these " vertical descents ", being at once more intelligent than cats and confronted with simpler problems. A parallel human situation to that of the cats would perhaps be that of a child tackling a stiff geometrical problem, and dimly recalling some parts of his solution and not others.

CHAPTER VI

1 See Chapter II above, p. 277.
2 *Educational Psychology*, by E. L. Thorndike, Vol. III, p. 387.
3 *Op. cit.*, p. 366.
4 *Op. cit.*, p. 367.
5 *Op. cit.*, pp. 363 and 364.
6 *Op. cit.*, p. 364.
7 *The Measurement of Intelligence* (1927), by E. L. Thorndike, p. 412.

8	*Op. cit.*, p. 20.	19	*Ibidem.*
9	*Op. cit.*, p. 25.	20	*Op. cit.*, p. 431.
10	*Op. cit.*, p. 59.	21	*Ibidem.*
11	*Op. cit.*, p. 481.	22	*Op. cit.*, p. 416.
12	*Op. cit.*, p. 422.	23	*Op. cit.*, p. 412.
13	*Op. cit.*, p. 427.	24	*Op. cit.*, p. 415.
14	*Op. cit.*, p. 430.	25	*Ibidem.*
15	*Ibidem.*	26	*Op. cit.*, p. 420.
16	*Op. cit.*, p. 415.	27	*Op. cit.*, p. 422.
17	*Op. cit.*, p. 420.	28	*Op. cit.*, p. 431.
18	*Op. cit.*, p. 421.		

29 *Brains of Rats and Men*, by C. J. Herrick, cf. p. 18.
30 A review of Spearman's *The Abilities of Man*, by P. M. Symonds, *Journal of Philosophy*, January 5, 1928.
31 *The Measurement of Intelligence*, by E. L. Thorndike, p. 19.
32 *Ibidem.*
33 *Ibidem.*
34 *Op. cit.*, p. 20.
35 *Ibidem.*

CHAPTER VII

1 See *The Nature of Intelligence and the Principles of Cognition*, by C. Spearman, cf. pp. 4, 5, 7. Also *The Abilities of Man*, by the same author, pp. 164-7.

2 It is fair to note that Spearman himself does not unreservedly identify intelligence with ' g,'. See *The Abilities of Man*, p. 412 : "Whether there is any advantage in attaching to this ' g ' the old mishandled label of intelligence seems at least dubious." On the other hand he claims ' g ' as a factor which enters into the measurement of ability of all kinds, and which is throughout constant for any individual, although varying greatly for different individuals. He finds that it is involved invariably and exclusively in all operations of an educative nature, whatever might be the class of relations or the sort of fundaments at issue ; also that it reveals a surprisingly complete independence of all manifestations of retentivity. If this is not intelligence, at any rate it has just the attributes of the faculty which we are attempting to discover. Moreover, Spearman himself tends at times to identify it with intelligence ; e.g. on p. 272 (*Abilities of man*) he asks, "Does a person's ' g ' (or intelligence) consist in his aptitude to acquire dispositions ? "

And on p. 350 of his *Nature of Intelligence*, after remarking that the term has lost any definite meaning in modern times and considering its equivalence to intellect (a special case of educing of relations, namely where the fundaments are highly abstract), he adds : " On the whole, however, circumstances appear to be driving us towards yet another alternative, which consists in extending the range of the word so as to cover all three noegenetic principles in every one of their manifestations." But the question at issue in the text is not as to the *term* but as to the fact (or faculty) Spearman's ' g ' as a three-process affair leaves us in doubt as to its underlying unity.

3 Spearman's hypothesis of a mental energy cannot be considered a satisfactory *psychological* answer. And would it not be an explanation of the known in terms of the less known ? See *Abilities of Man*, Chapter IX.

4 *Abilities of Man*, p. 195.

5 *The Nature of Intelligence*, etc., p. 48.

6 *Op. cit.*, p. 63.

7 *Op. cit.*, p. 91.

8 *The Abilities of Man*, p. 3.

9 *Mentality of Apes*, by W. Kohler, p. 49.

10 *The Measurement of Intelligence*, by L. M. Terman, p. 243.

11 *The Nature of Intelligence*, etc., by C. Spearman, p. 112.

12 The interested reader may care to examine some of the

following definitions and descriptions of intelligence with a view to determine of each :

a. How far the author pre-supposes the word to cover a *general mental efficiency*, or a *particular capacity* separate from memory, imagination, affection, conation, etc., yet determining the intelligence of all behaviour.

b. Whether what holds true in the definition or description does so in virtue of the common psychological factor described in our text :

(1) The capacity to solve problems (Allport, Claparede).

(2) The capacity for knowledge (Henman).

(3) The power of progressing in representative learning (Dearborn).

(4) General mental adaptibility to new problems and conditions of life (W. Stern).

(5) Mental balance (Freeman).

(6) The facility with which old responses can be hitched on to new situations (Thomson).

(7) Voluntary attention is the essential factor of general intelligence. " A capacity for continually systematizing mental behaviour by forming new psycho-physical co-ordinations, older co-ordinations being retained " (Burt).

(8) Ability to take and retain a given mental set.
    Power of auto-criticism.
    Ability to make adaptations for the purpose of attaining a desired end (Binet).

(9) The ability for independent and creative thinking (Meumann).

(10) Comprehending in a unitary whole impressions independent and partly contradictory (Ebbinghaus).

(11) Something which sees more than the senses convey, which reasons upon what it sees, which invests it with an idea (Cardinal Newman).

(12) A faculty of manufacturing artificial objects, especially tools to make tools, and of indefinitely varying the manufacture (Bergson).

(13) A biological mechanism by which the effects of a complexity of stimuli are brought together and given a somewhat unified effect in behaviour (J. Peterson).

CHAPTER VIII

1 From *Habit and Instinct*, by C. Lloyd Morgan ; cited by W. McDougall in *Outline of Psychology*, p. 74.

2 *Outline of Psychology*, by W. McDougall, p. 110.

3 *Instincts and Habits of the Solitary Wasps*, by G. W. and E. G. Peckham, pp. 40 and 232.

4 *Mentality of Apes*, by W. Köhlcr, pp. 21 and 291.

5 *Op. cit.*, Peckham, p. 22.

6 See *The Great Society*, by Graham Wallas, pp. 40-56 ; and " Thinking as an Instinct," by E. F. Heidbreder, *Psychological Review*, Vol. 33, 1926, pp. 279-97.

7 *Social Psychology*, by W. McDougall, p. 58.

CHAPTER IX

1 *Social Psychology*, by W. McDougall, p. 44.

2 *Problems of Personality* by various authors ; article on " Character and Inhibition," by A. A. Roback (esp. pp. 79-138 and 115-22). See also *The Psychology of Character*, by A. A. Roback, pp. 485-8.

3 *Problems of Personality*, p. 134. " It is within reason, I think, to postulate a consistency urge as the basis of all conduct typifying the person of character. Like other connate tendencies, this urge requires sufficient time for maturation. Young children seldom give indications of this tendency, yet it is possible to detect significant differences in reactions to others on the part of even five-year-old youngsters, and that in spite of their being brought up in the same environment."

4 *Op. cit.*, p. 131.

5 *Outline of Psychology*, by W. McDougall, pp. 417-50. Also *Outline of Abnormal Psychology* (same author), pp. 525 *seq.*

6 *Outline of Psychology*, p. 442.

7 McDougall himself recognizes this harmony (*Outline of Psychology*, p. 446) : " Will is character in action ; and in our most complete volitions, following upon deliberation, the intellect co-operates fully with character." It is the motive suggested by McDougall, namely satisfaction of an ideal spectator, that is in question.

CHAPTER X

1 Instances, taken almost at random, from writers whose works are for the most part in general use, and who explain away Volition or postpone treatment of it to the end of their books (or both) are : Breese (*Psychology*), Cameron (*Educational Psychology*), Carr (*Psychology*), Gates (*Educational Psychology and Elements of Psychology*), Gault and Howard (*Outlines of General Psychology*), McDougall (*Outline of Psychology*), Pillsbury (*Fundamentals of Psychology*), Thorndike (*Educational Psychology*),

Warren (*Human Psychology* and *Elements of Human Psychology*),
Woodworth (*Psychology, a Study of Mental Life*). Though James
discusses the will at length, he does not consider it, except
incidentally, till towards the end of his second volume, after he has
built up his system on a manly sensationist, and if we push him
to it, a deterministic basis. Thorndike has no considered treatment of will at all in his Educational Psychology ; he refers to it
occasionally in disparaging terms.

2 See, for a clear and brief criticism of this view of will, *The
Elements of Social Justice*, by L. T. Hobhouse ; Chapter III on
" Moral Freedom," esp. p. 53.

3 Psychologists of different schools resort to a " whole self "
rendering of will ; e.g.

Pierre Janet : " The will depends on the totality of the
tendencies."

W. McDougall : " Will is character in action ; and in the most
complete Volition, following upon deliberation, the intellect
co-operates fully with character. Volition thus becomes the
expression of the whole personality."

H. C. Warren : " The prominent feature of voluntary control
is that the action is determined by the man's whole life, not merely
by present situation."

H. Bergson : " We are free when our acts emanate from our
entire personality."

F. Paulhan : " It is rather for the action which engages more
completely the aggregate of personality that we reserve the name
of willing."

L. T. Hobhouse : " Moral freedom, then, has nothing to do
with isolation, but is, as has been said, the harmony of the whole
self in the multitudinous relations which constitute the web of
its interests."

Perhaps the attractiveness and part of the plausibility of the
" whole self " or " entire personality " dogma lies in its adapt-
ability of meaning to the taste of the individual psychologist, e.g.

a. An ensemble of impulses (Gault and Howard).

b. The outcome of one's whole past (Pillsbury and Warren).

c. A harmony of principle with practice (Hobhouse and
McDougall).

d. The resultant of careful all-round deliberation (Woodworth).

It seems better to abandon a phrase susceptible of so many
interpretations.

Another reason for the plausibility of the phrase is in the
suggestion it contains of universality of some kind—it has a
scientific smack about it.

4 *Fundamentals of Psychology*, by W. B. Pillsbury, pp. 534 on.

5 *Psychology, a Study of Mental Life*, by R. S. Woodworth, p. 533.

6 *Principles of Psychology*, by W. James, Vol. II, p. 531 *seq.*, and his briefer course, pp. 429 on.

7 *Outline of General Psychology*, by R. H. Gault and D. T. Howard, p. 374. "We prefer to mean by the term will an ensemble of impulses ; or better, the energy of the organism which is released in the sensory impulse, in perception, in con- ceptual thought, in attention and released by our contacts of every sort with our changing surroundings."

The citation is given not because of any special authority attaching to it, but as illustrative of the kind of interpretation of " the whole man " to which a mechanistic psychology is driven.

8 To the possible mechanistic rejoinder that on analysis every new response will be found to be only a new combination of old responses there are two answers :

a. It is not true. The boy learning to sharpen his pencil is acquiring refinements of movement, and the student learning history new items of information, the scientist making a new discovery new knowledge, which he has not acquired or even been capable of before.

b. In the kind of way in which it appears to hold, e.g. in com- bining notes already separately known to form a new piece of music, of colours already familiar to form a new picture, or words already known to form a new story, etc., the fact is that the newness does not consist in the aggregate of old notes or letters or words or what not, but in the mind's contribution to the result. There is always apprehension of relations or reproduction of what has been apprehended, or more generally, if not quite generally, both apprehension and reproduction, of relations and inter- relations between objects of thought.

9 For a distinction between conation and volition, see " The Psychology of Conation and Volition," by F. P. Aveling, *British Journal Psychology*, 1926, Vol. XVI. He represents volition as distinct from conation, as consciousness of self. There is a strengthening of motive by reference to or adoption by the self.

See also " Experimental Study on the Mental Processes Involved in Judgment," by B. P. Stevanovic, *British Journal Psychology*, *Monthly Supplement XII* (1927). His evidence shows there may be volition but no conation in judging ; and that conation, but not volition, is objectively indicated by bodily changes recorded by the psycho-galvanic reflex.

Similarly, in her experimental study on " The Phenomenology of Acts of Choice," *British Journal Psychology, Monthly Supple- ment XI* (1927) H. M. Wells finds evidence of a clear distinction between consciousness of striving and consciousness of self, and stresses that consciousness of self-activity appears in voluntary choice ; a consciousness which is keenest in hard choices, where the self vigorously adopts an unpleasant alternative.

CHAPTER XI

1 See " In Defence of Behaviourism," by J. B. Watson, *Psyche*, July, 1924, p. 11. " Now when we see a child reacting with his arms and legs, duplicating his father's morning exercises, we feel that there is no mystery about such actions. Again, when we hear him talking, the act seems simple and straightforward. But when we see the child sitting quietly for two minutes and then hear him suddenly exclaim : " Daddy, I just thought about the party I went to with you yesterday," we fall down in worship. " My child has begun to think ! " Thinking is a mysterious process which can never be studied, only *venerated*. To the behaviourist the process of thinking is not mysterious. May I say it is as simple and straightforward as tennis playing ? "

For Thorndike's attitude see note 4, Chapter XIII below, pp. 314 *ff*.

2 The removal of mystery from any single fact or object is beyond human capacity. Until recently physicists took it for granted that investigations into basic entities (force, energy, mass, space, time, etc.) were giving some special access to the inner secret of being ; and further that somehow the mystery of the universe (at any rate on its material, if not also on its spiritual side) might be cleared up by disclosing some exceedingly minute common somethings (call them atoms or electrons or what not) of which it was built up. It is at last being realized that

a. There is no special self-evidence or absence of mystery in being very small ;

b. Even if we do ever arrive at a common something we still do not know its inner nature ; and

c. We cannot tell why the particular complications and combinations of that something which constitute its larger manifestations to the naked eye are what they are or behave as they behave or have the effects they do have.

Professor A. S. Eddington, in an article on " The Domain of Physical Science " in *Science, Religion, and Reality* (edited by J. Needham), writes : " Physics is now in course of abandoning its claim to a type of knowledge which it formerly asserted without hesitation." Physics, he tells us, merely describes a series of inter-dependent relations without giving any explanation of what is being explained—the various basic entities of physics, motion, energy, mass, etc., are described in terms of one another, a circular argument. " The chain of connection of the entities of the world is the province of physics, but the intrinsic essence of these entities is now recognized to be outside its province."

Op. cit., p. 206 : " The nineteenth century physicist thought he knew what matter was, namely, atoms. But now physics has nothing to say as to the ultimate nature of an atom ; what it studies is the linkage of atomic properties to other terms in the physicist's vocabulary, each depending on the others in endless chain with the same inscrutable nature running through the whole."

We have thus no more hope of removing the mystery from being (whether living or non-living) by reducing it to electron-protons than by referring it to some spiritual origin or cause.

3 It is significant that physicists have lately taken to questioning the absolute uniformity and the determinateness of apparently uniform physical phenomena. To-day the atom is regarded (by Whitehead and others) not as a mechanism, but as an organism. " Science is taking on a new aspect which . . . is neither purely physical nor purely biological. It is becoming a study of organisms. Biology is the study of larger organisms, whereas physics is a study of the smaller organisms." The latest picture of the atom contains no mark or factor to decide what *that* atom will do next (although it contains factors deciding the average conduct of a large number of such atoms). Thus the apparent determinism of physics is now found to be merely high probability. See A. S. Eddington's Gifford Lectures as reported in *Nature*, February 26, 1927 ; and *Philosophy*, by Bertrand Russell, Chapter XIV, on pp. 144 *sqq.*

4 Two meanings of the term cause should be distinguished :

a. The temporarily prior of two events ; more specifically, that of two events which is first in time, and without which the second would not occur ;

b That which makes an event occur.

Contrast, for example, the impact of a billiard ball causing the movement of another (cause in the first sense) with my producing a poem or building a house (cause in the second). By analogy, the initiative (the power to make happen) of the animate being is read into the first of the two inanimate events, an unwarranted anthropomorphization, giving rise to the concept of force, and blind force, because unintelligent and unconscious. But though we may rightly regard such a cause as a mental fiction, we are not thereby justified in discarding cause in the sense of human and animal initiative. Popularly also the term cause is sometimes loosely used of

(1) Material components or constituents. A movement of the air is the cause of wind, or a gathering of people the cause of a crowd.

(2) An end more or less consciously entertained. A war is caused by international jealousies ; or the choice of a career by one's ambition or one's desire for money.

In all cases the one underlying common element is that without which the fact, effect, or event would not have occurred.

As regards the argument in the text the points to note are that the only cause that we know directly (in our own volition, as a fact of immediate experience) and therefore demanding no further proof is cause in the sense of making an event happen ; and that where the term is used in any of the other senses, we have no right to embody in it without proof the former meaning also. But there is a natural tendency through verbal association to do so.

5 The recognition of an ultimate or prime cause, it should be noted, really lands us in indeterminism ; for either that first cause is itself caused, in which case it is not ultimate and the premise is contradicted, or it is not caused, in which case it is the arbitrary or at least the undetermined initiator of the chain of events.

6 See e.g. *Riddles of the Sphinx*, by F. C. S. Schiller, p. 73. " Originally . . . the conception of cause was a transference of the internal sense of volition and effort to things outside the organism. The changes in the world were supposed to be due to the action of immanent spirits. In course of time these divine spirits were no longer regarded as directly causing events, but as being the first causes which set secondary causes in motion. It was then supposed that cause and effect were connected as by chains of necessity, which ultimately depended from the first cause of them all."

In *Philosophy* (p. 115), Bertrand Russell writes : " We must not have any notion of ' compulsion ' as if the cause* forced the effect to happen. . . . Compulsion is anthropomorphism ; a man is compelled to do something when he wishes to do the opposite, but except where human or animal wishes come in, the notion of compulsion is inapplicable.   Science is concerned merely with what happens, not with what must happen."

7 See *The Persistent Problems of Philosophy*, by M. W. Calkins, p. 129. " We know too little of the relation between cause and effect to assert dogmatically that the two must be of the same nature.   In fact, among observed cases of causality the difference

*As antecedent event.

between cause and effect is often very striking, as when mechanical causes produce thermal effects, or electrical causes physiological effects."

If this holds of cause in the sense of invariable (or customary) antecedent, it holds even more clearly of cause as mediator or initiator of an event. I am not the same as the building or poem or movement I create. The modern doctrine of emergent evolution stresses the unpredictable differences between effects and causes.

8 Three recent doctrines—the Gestalt in psychology, and those of emergence and relativity in physical science—agree in emphasizing the effectual differences involved in rearrangements of *prima face* identical constituents. To the Gestalt psychologist every item in a whole takes its character from the configuration or pattern as a whole ; to the emergent evolutionist H_2O is very different from the sum of its constituents H_2 and O : (nor could these differences have been deduced or predicted) ; while according to the doctrine of relativity (if I understand it so far) the particular spatio-temporal relations which obtain in any case make all the difference in the world (or in the universe) to the event concerned.

CHAPTER XII

Psychic Dominants

1 Instances of psychic dominants in the past, which the public mind has outgrown, are easy to recognize, e.g. the Ptolemaic cosmology which, coupled with the theological conviction of the central importance of man, prevented acceptance of the Copernican system ; the mediaeval ' preconceived perfection ' which was used as an argument for discrediting the discovery of sunspots, and even against Harvey's discovery of the circulation of the blood, a constant return of the blood to the heart being regarded as an imperfect arrangement ; on the same principle an Italian surgeon was condemned by the ecclesiastical authorities for his plastic operations to repair defects of nose, ear and lips ; and even in quite recent times the same notion underlies opposition to vaccination and the use of anæsthetics in childbirth as interfering with the arrangements of nature or of God. The theological dominants which prevented (and still in benighted areas prevent) the acceptance of the principles of evolution are well known.

A particular example was the effect of the calculation of a seventeenth century archbishop that Adam lived 4,004 years before Christ, thus making the earth some 6,000 years old. " The adoption of this belief had a retarding effect upon the development of general geological ideas for nearly two centuries ; for any attempt to explain the accumulation and deformation of rocks in so short a period had of necessity to introduce supernatural convulsions, or to assume all rocks were formed in the course of a few days in the condition and situation in which they now occur. Nearly all the eminent thinkers of that period were influenced by that belief, which gave rise to the fantastic theories of the earth to which reference has already been made." (From " An Episode in the History of Geology," by F. J. North, *Discovery*, May, 1928, p. 157).

Each generation criticizes the unconscious assumptions made by its parents, but is in turn unconscious of its own, until they again are in the face of opposition brought to light. Yet error never can be refuted till it has been clearly envisaged ; and " an unformulated and unrefuted error may work incalculable injury from the shadowy recesses of the mind which vaguely holds it."

A point to note about the effect of these dominants is that people subject to them are apt to accept readily what accords, but to exact excessive evidence for what does not accord, with the unconscious dominant view. For example owing to the pseudo-scientific dominant (that science, the organised search for truth, can admit only invariable uniformities whether the universe is ' uniform ' or not) we find psychologists assuming that volition is illusory until it is proved valid (since it seems to upset such uniformities), but that sense percepts in general are valid unless they are proved illusory.

Again one even hears it claimed by those subject to the materialistic dominant (that ultimate reality must be some tangible perceptible *thing*) that consciousness itself does not exist, no proof of it being apparently regarded as sufficient. Hence science must take note only of overt behaviour. As if a judge would refuse to accept the evidence of witnesses until they first proved they were alive.

The ' psychic dominant ' has a serious negative influence : it blinds its victims to familiar and obvious phenomena around them. Charles Darwin remarks the peculiar blindness of Sedgwick the geologist and himself when geologizing in the Welsh hills : " We spent many hours in Crum Idwal examining all the rocks with extreme care, as Sedgwick was anxious to find fossils in them ; but neither of us saw a trace of the wonderful glacial phenomena all around us ; we did not notice the plainly scored rocks, the perched boulders, the lateral and terminal moraines. Yet these phenomena are so conspicuous that, as I afterwards declared in the philosophical magazine, a house burnt down by fire did not tell its story more plainly than did that valley."

Just as geology dominated by its interest in fossils and facts, evidences of the creative enterprise of the Almighty, was blind to a tale writ large on every side, so modern psychology keeps turning a blind eye to plain evidences of volitional activity on every side, because it is subject to the psychic dominant of mechanism.

2 The objector may ask how this self-activity takes place ; and imply that if we cannot provide an answer self-activity is to be discredited. To the question how this activity takes place there is no answer, any more than one can say how it comes about that H plus O produces H2O or how certain flowers produce the particular fragrance known as violet. All we can do is to describe certain conditions or accompaniments of the event, leaving the event itself a mystery. Our investigation of the ways in which human activity originates shows that some activities we originate in accordance with innate urges ; and some apart from or even in defiance of innate urges ; and some (reflexes) *we* do not seem to originate at all ; they happen to us. To the pure volitionist the last named, to the pure mechanist the second may seem the more mysterious, and to demand a further ' how.' But in all three cases we are up against inexplicables.

The inability to explain how a mental power acts cannot be accepted as a disproof that it does act : our inability to explain how the golf champion made his strokes does not prove that he did not make them.

3 We may repeat that self-activity is not unique in being unique, or *sui generis.* Equally mysterious, equally *sui generis,* as far as we can discover, are electrons and protons, or whatever form of elemental being underlies the various physical basic entities.

Recent science recognizes the atom which once seemed so intelligible an ultimate basis of matter—requiring no further explanation—as itself comprising or constituted of, units of energy (of positive and negative electricity) of which the electrons are billions of times smaller than an atom, and resembling in important respects (on its, to us, tiny scale) the vast solar, and still more immense sidereal, systems. " From the point of view of an electron an atom is a big thing with plenty of room inside it ; it is mostly empty space, like the solar system." There is nothing more ultimately intelligible about an atom (250 millions of which in a row would stretch something like an inch) than about the milky way or about our being able to think about these things. There are no ultimate causes and no ultimate specks of matter in which the human mind as we know it can come to rest.

(See *Modern Scientific Ideas,* by Sir Oliver Lodge, or *The Atom,* by E. N. da C. Andrade).

4 In *The Foundations of Character* A. Shand describes the development of character in terms of emotions and sentiments or systems of emotional·tendencies. He acknowledges that in isolating the emotions and sentiments " we shall in a certain sense personify them," but adds, " such a personification does not falsify their nature so long as we do not attribute to them qualities which they do not possess—so long as we do not confuse them with the total self to which they belong." (p. 65).

Yet in his summary treatment " of the will and intelligence in relation to character " (*op. cit.*, ch. VI, pp. 64-7) this is precisely the fallacy he proceeds to commit. He identifies strong and weak wills with strength and weakness of innate tendencies : " those who seem born to rule and those who are naturally submissive ; those who exercise great self-control and those who are impulsive." Thus he endows impulse (according to him, one of the constituents of emotion) with volition. Innate impulse swallows will, e.g. " It may reasonably be urged that the will is not an independent force—at least in the beginning, or before it develops the power of real choice ; that it is an expression of the tendencies of emotions and sentiments ; that in them its innate qualities are manifested, and its acquired qualities developed." Again : " Strength or weakness of will, other things equal, varies with the strength or weakness of the emotions or sentiment to which it belongs." " Every strong sentiment has a tendency to develop a strong will in its support." " The strength or weakness of the will is largely due to the sentiment in which it is organized, or to the direct influence of emotion." (From our point of view the reverse is true. Volition is expressed in control of emotion and sentiment, not as an expression of them). But Shand has certain qualms about his attitude. He goes on : " But if we do seem to choose between sentiments ; and if there is our one self separate from our many selves—the sum of the dispositions of our emotions and sentiments, then if this be the fact, it is not the kind of fact which we can take into account. The science of character will be the science of our sentiments and emotions—of these many selves, not of this one self."

(Is it the pseudo-scientific dominant that induces Shand to decide to ignore an important truth *even if it be true* ?)

His treatment of intelligence is similar. " The science of character will deal with Intellect as with the Will. It will regard the one no more than the other as an independent existence ; but as organized in and subserving the system of some impulse, emotion, or sentiment." But again if there be sometimes manifested in us " a pure Intelligence, free from all admixture of emotion or sentiment . . . if this be a fact, a science of character cannot deal with it."

Thus Shand regards science as the search for truth *on terms*, that is on the condition of its squaring with his preconception of what he expects truth to be ; and thus too he disposes of will and intelligence by embodying them inside emotion or sentiments.

A few quotations from Thorndike's *Educational Psychology* must suffice to indicate his aggrandisement of the neurones, (Vol. i, p. 311) : " The original nature of man, as we have seen, has its source far back of reason and morality in the interplay of brute forces : it grows up as an agency to keep men and especially certain neurones within men's bodies, alive ; it is physiologically determined by the character of the synaptic bonds and degrees of readiness to act of these neurones . . . amongst the neurones whose life it serves are neurones whose life means, if a certain social environment is provided, loving children, being just to all men, seeking the truth, and every other activity that man shows. . . ." (Here the neurones absorb emotions, and apparently have the intelligence to discriminate one social environment from another).

On p. 298 we read that superior interest in the forces, needs, and beauties of nature " is the readiness of certain neurones to act, manifested as the satisfyingness of certain states of affairs to her " (that is to the observer, in this case Miss Calkins). (Thus apparently the neurones have æsthetic discrimination).

P. 228 : " The learning of an animal is an instinct of its neurones " (i.e. the neurones are naturally intelligent). P. 226 : " For this con-ductive process in the neurones to be interfered with in a given state of affairs is the physiological fact that we mean when we say that the state of affairs is annoying." (Thus anger is not aroused by conscious cognition, but by whether our physical nerves are working in one way or in another).

P. 170 : " It is a fact of original nature that certain states of affairs are satisfying to a man's neurones—are such that as they do nothing to avoid, whereas other states of affairs are annoying to the neurones—stimulate them to do something until the annoying state of affairs gives way to a satisfying one which they do nothing to avoid."

(Thorndike ' puts it over' the unwary student, when he comes to his educational applications of the doctrine of satisfaction and annoyance, by confusing this colourless satisfaction and annoyance of the neurones with the conscious emotional states of satisfaction and annoyance of the whole individual).

P. 11 : " The history of modern explanations of human intellect, character, and skill shows three notable stages. In the

S

first certain mythical potencies were postulated which when aroused to action by the events of a man's life produced his thought and acts. These potencies were ' instinct ' which could do almost everything in (sic) a pinch, the ' will ', and the faculties —memory, attention, reasoning, and the like."

(Here volition is refused admission on its merits, as a mythical potency.)

Vol. 2, p. 23 : Man " is first of all an association mechanism, working to avoid what disturbs the life processes of certain neurones. If we begin by fabricating imaginary powers and faculties, or if we avoid thought by loose and empty terms, or if we stay lost in wonder at the extraordinary versatility and inventiveness of the higher forms of learning, we shall never understand man's progress or control his education."

(Thus we see from these two citations that while the neurones are not supposed to be mysterious the higher thought processes are. To put the neurones in charge is to make wonder superfluous).

Vol. 2, p. 19 : " Other cases follow the same simple association plan, save that *ideas* are the terms in the association series." (Here the neurones swallow intelligence. They have ideas). Vol. 2, p. 53 : " That the set or attitude of the man helps to determine which bonds shall satisfy and which shall annoy has commonly been somewhat obscured by vague assertions that the selection and retention is of what is ' in point ' or is ' the right one ' or is ' appropriate ' or the like. It is thus asserted or at least hinted that ' the will ', ' the voluntary attention ', ' the consciousness of the problem ', and other such entities are endowed with magic power to decide what is the ' right ' or ' useful ' bond and to kill off the others."

(Intelligence is thus explained away in terms of neuronic combinations, which thus embody it).

5   It will be objected that everybody espouses some philosophy or other : it is implied in his particular opinions and conduct, even though he has not made his principles explicit to himself. The mere moneymaker implies for example a belief in material values, the philanthropist in other-worldliness, etc.

The claim made in the text however is not that the ardent pursuer of science or anybody else implies in his pursuits no system of beliefs and valuations—I do not mean by " espousing no philosophy ' that we must act on no beliefs or entertain no values ; but that as scientists, in regard to the science we are pursuing scientifically, we must not begin by accepting pre- suppositions about the ultimate nature of its subject matter or of the truths which our study will yield us. Our first duty is to consider the data as we find them, and to avoid, as far as we can, coming to them with a set of preconceptions or dogmas taken from elsewhere. To approach the science of psychology already committed say to a spiritualistic interpretation of the universe is just as unscientific as to approach it with a mechanistic bent.

As creatures of our time and place it is of course impossible for even the most detached of us to approach any subject at every moment quite impartially, but it is just in the care taken to view the data of our science as they present themselves directly to consciousness, and to avoid twisting them (by force of unconscious habit) to fit this or that psychic dominant, that the scientific spirit resides. Only on these terms can we expect to present for further synthesis to the philosopher the facts of the case as we find them in our particular field ; otherwise we handicap him by prejudging his conclusions for him. We ensnare him in a vicious circle.

To espouse no philosophy, then, does not mean to imply no generalities at all, but to strive to let the data imply their own. This we can do only by steering clear of ultimate presuppositions as much as possible, by letting each fact as it appears tell its own story ; and by building up our provisional principles accordingly.

My own contention is that if we so approach the data of psychology we shall find both mechanism and volition ; and our provisional principles will make room for both.

6 See *Philosophy*, by Bertrand Russell, p. 144.

" The old view was that an event A will always be followed by a certain event B, and that the problem of discovering causal laws is the problem, given an event B, of finding that event A which is its invariable antecedent or vice versa. At an early stage of a science this point of view is useful ; it gives laws which are true usually, though probably not always, and it affords the basis for more exact laws. But it has no philosophical validity, and is superseded in science as soon as we arrive at genuine laws. Genuine laws, in advanced sciences, are practically always quantitative laws of *tendency*." He goes on to illustrate from the atom of which we have statistical knowledge of the behaviour of its constituent electrons. " Now at some moment . . . the electron in our atom jumps to a smaller orbit, and the energy lost to the atom travels outward in a light-wave. We know no causal law as to when the electron will jump, though we know how far it will jump and exactly what will happen in the neighbourhood when it does. At least when I say we know exactly what will happen, I ought to say that we know exactly the mathematical laws of what will happen."

CHAPTER XIII

1 *Human and Animal Behaviour*, W. Wundt, pp. 224 *sqq.*

2 *Ibidem*, pp. 299 *sqq.*

3 *Ibidem*, p. 232. " The chief motive of actual volitions is henceforth not some particular sense impression which happens to be there, but the entire trend of consciousness as determined by its previous experiences."
" The action which results from this plurality of conflicting motives we call a complex voluntary action or a volitional action."

4 *Ibidem*, pp. 432 *sqq.* : Discussion of the nature of the Personal Factor. In volitional action personality or character (the inmost nature of personality) is the only immediate cause of action, ' motives ' being only the mediate causes of them. " As long as there remain individuals who resist this force [namely of the social environment] we shall be obliged to take into account a personal factor if we are to understand the causality of the particular voluntary action." Yet " The determinants of volition which have their source in the social condition of the people come within the causal nexus of natural and historical processes. They serve then to prove once and for all that the will is not undetermined." Again, " The motives which determine the will are parts of the universal chain of natural causation." Thus Wundt lands on the determinist side of the fence.

5 *Psychology*, by William James (Briefer Course), pp. 5, 16, 457.

6 *Ibidem.* pp. 415, 416.

7 *Ibidem*, pp. 419 and 420.

8 *Ibidem*, p. 415.

9 *Ibidem*, p. 427.

10 *Ibidem*, p. 420.

11 *Ibidem*, p. 426.

12 *Ibidem*, p. 457.

13 *Ibidem*, pp. 448 *sqq.*

14 *Ibidem*, p. 455.

15 *Ueber den Willensakt und der Temperament*, by N. Ach.

16 *Ibidem*, p. 241.

17 *Etude Experimentale sur les Choix Voluntaire*, by A. Michotte and E. Prüm.

18 *Motive Force and Motivation Tracks*, by Boyd Barrett.

19 *An Experimental Investigation of the Process of Choosing*, by R. H. Wheeler (University of Oregon Publications).

20 *Psychical Review*, 1921, pp. 356 *sqq.* ; 1922, pp. 425 *sqq.* *American Journal of Psychology*, 1915, pp. 459 *sqq.*

21 *The Phenomenolgy of Acts of Choice*, by H. Wells (*British Journal of Psychology Monograph Supplement*, 11).

22 *Ibidem*, p. 135.

Referring to Wheeler's contentions she concludes :

" We find no justification for Wheeler's statement that consciousness of ' self-activity ' can be analyzed into the basal elements of kinaesthetic and organic sensations and images. We find that consciousness of ' self-activity ' is absolutely distinct and different from the kinaesthetic and organic phenomena which may or may not be present with it. In our opinion if there is anything ' basal ' in consciousness, certainly ' action ' is ; and further it is unanalyzable. In maintaining that action states are interpretations of sensations and images, Wheeler is really affirming a ' faculty ' of interpretation which makes it possible for them to occur." (p. 147.)

INDEX

Ach : 232, 268
Allport, F. H. : 14ff, 248
Association, and Intelligence : 60ff
  and Stupidity : 65
  Ambiguous meanings of : 67
  and Relation : 68
Attention : 230ff
Autonomic activities : 18
Aveling, F. P. : 257

Bernard, L. C. : 14, 19ff, 248
Binet : 9, 12
Boyd Barrett : 234, 268

Calkins : 235, 260
Carr, W. : 247
Cause : 153, 160, 169ff, 259ff
  and effect : 170ff
Character : 124, 244ff
Colvin : 15
Choice, object of : 209
  consciousness of : 207, 215
Conation : 148, 155, 257
  and volition : 155ff, 257
Conduct and intelligence : 127ff
Configuration : 32ff ; *see also*
  Gestalt
Consciousness : 16ff, 73, 162, 248,
  249
  economy of : 48
  levels of : 53ff, 104, 108, 109
  of freedom : 206
  of choice : 207, 215
Conscience : 122
Curiosity and Intelligence : 113

Eddington : 258
Emotion : 14, 17, 24
  and instinct : 103

Faculty psychology : 6-8, 201ff
Free Will : 136ff, 153 (*see also*
  Volition)
" Fiat " : 220ff

Gestalt, Ch. IV. : 38ff, 83, 154,
  238 n., 261

Habit : 239ff
Herrick, C. J. : 252
Hobhouse, L. T. : 256
Hypostatization : 183ff, 198, 264,
  265

Ideo-motor theory : 220ff, 231
Illusion : 193ff
Impulse(s), nature of : 40
  in instinct : 102ff
  and will : 139ff, 202ff
  conflict of : 208ff
  and principle : 211ff
Imageless thought : 226ff
Inhibition : 124
Initiative : 144, 148, 153ff, 165,
  170, 221
Insight : 32ff, 38ff, 54
Instinct : 15, 240
  and intelligence : 6, Ch. VIII.
  Symposium on : 11
  and emotion : 103
  human and insect : 103
Intelligence, reasons for neglect
  of : Ch. I
  faculty of : 43, 80
  symposium on : 11
  definition of : 11, 19, 22,
    26ff, 29, 58, 59, 93ff, 250,
    254
  as successful trials : 18, 20ff
  and initiative : 19ff
  as adjustment : 21, 94
  and " drive " : 23
  and urge : 26ff
  of apes : 32, 34ff, 89, 105,
    108, 118
  and repetition : 35
  tests of : 8ff
  criterion of : 10, 29, 38, 82
  nature of : 42ff, 68, 92, 112
  verbal ambiguity : 43ff
  and mental efficiency : 44
  grades of : 54, 56, 63, 74,
    77ff, 96, 110, 151
  and memory · 45, 55
  and creative imagination : 56

271

multiple theory of : 59ff
and association : 60ff
and training : 70
physiological view of : 70ff
and conation : 86
as integration : 88
and conceptual thinking : 96
and instinct, Ch. VIII.
and mechanism : 109
as instinctive : 111ff
and curiosity : 113
and impulse : 120ff
and principle : 126ff
and conduct : 127ff
and volition : Ch. X.
and " g " : Ch. VII., 253
Introspection : 4, 232

James : 142, Ch. XIII, 251, 268

Koffka : 32ff, 251
Köhler : 32ff, 89, 105, 108, 118, 251, 253

Learning : 43ff, 95
animal and human : 46
scope of : 46
repetitions and variations in : 47
Loeb, J. : 247

McDougall : 15, 103, 113, 115–120, 125, 247, 254, 255
Mechanism and Intelligence : 109
Mechanistic psychology : 6, 24, 123, 154, 219
explanations : 70, 160, 166ff, 265ff
Memory : 22, 44, 242
Meumann : 12
Michotte : 233, 268
Morgan, Lloyd : 5, 247
Motive, fallacy of the single : 212
Myers, C. S. : 247, 250

Noegenesis : 82ff

Parsimony, canon of : 5, 247
Peckham : 255
Peterson, J. : 247
Pillsbury : 139, 256
Play : 116
Predictability : 149
Prüm : 233, 268
Psychological Science : 176ff

Psychology, science of : 4ff, 134ff, 149, Ch. XI., 176, 218
animal : 5
mechanistic *(see* Mechanistic)
faculty in : 7, 200ff
function in : 8
physiological : 4, 19ff, 135
and ethics : 192ff
Physical Science : 24, 258ff
Psychic dominants : 176ff, 261ff
Psycho-physical parallelism : 72

Reflex, conditioned : 16, 248
Reflex(es) : 15ff, 219
Repetition : 171, 190, 219, 221, 241, 257
Rignano : 251
Roback : 124
Romanes : 5, 247
Rüger, H. A. : 251
Russell, Bertrand : 259, 267

Schiller, F. C. S. : 260
Science *(see* Psychology) : 160ff
and mystery : 161ff
and universal law : 163ff
Scientific explanation : 182
psychology : 218
Self activity : 144, 180, 233ff, 242 *(see* Volition)
Sentiment : 125, 183ff
Shand : 183, 264
Spearman : Ch. VII., 253
Specialist bias : 233ff
Stern : 12
Stevanovic : 257
Stimulus, subordinate to urge : 26
Stimulus Response : 13ff, 58ff, 154
definitions of : 248
Stout : 247

Terman : 90, 253
Thinking : 16, 26ff
Thorndike : 5, 32, 46, 53, 55, Ch. VI., 93, 152, 183, 247, 251ff, 265
Thurstone : Ch. III., 250
Trial and Error : 16, 27, 29ff, 32, 52ff, 154, 249

Unitary Factor : 43, 59ff, 80

Variation : 171 *(see also* Repetition)

Vitalism : 185
Volition : 121ff
  and intelligence : Ch. X.
  grades of : 151, 191, 204ff
  and conation : 155ff
  and law : 163ff
  uniqueness of : Ch. XII.
  and imagery : 220ff
  and attention : 230ff
  experiments on : 231ff
  (*see also* Free Will)

Wallas, Graham : 255
Warden, C. J. : 247
Watson : 17, 247, 248, 258
Weiss, A. P. : 247
Wells, H. M. : 235ff, 268
Wheeler, R. H. : 234ff, 268
Will, Strength of : 158
  definitions of : 256 (*see also*
    Volition)
Woodworth : 22, 141, 257
Wundt : Ch. XIII, 268